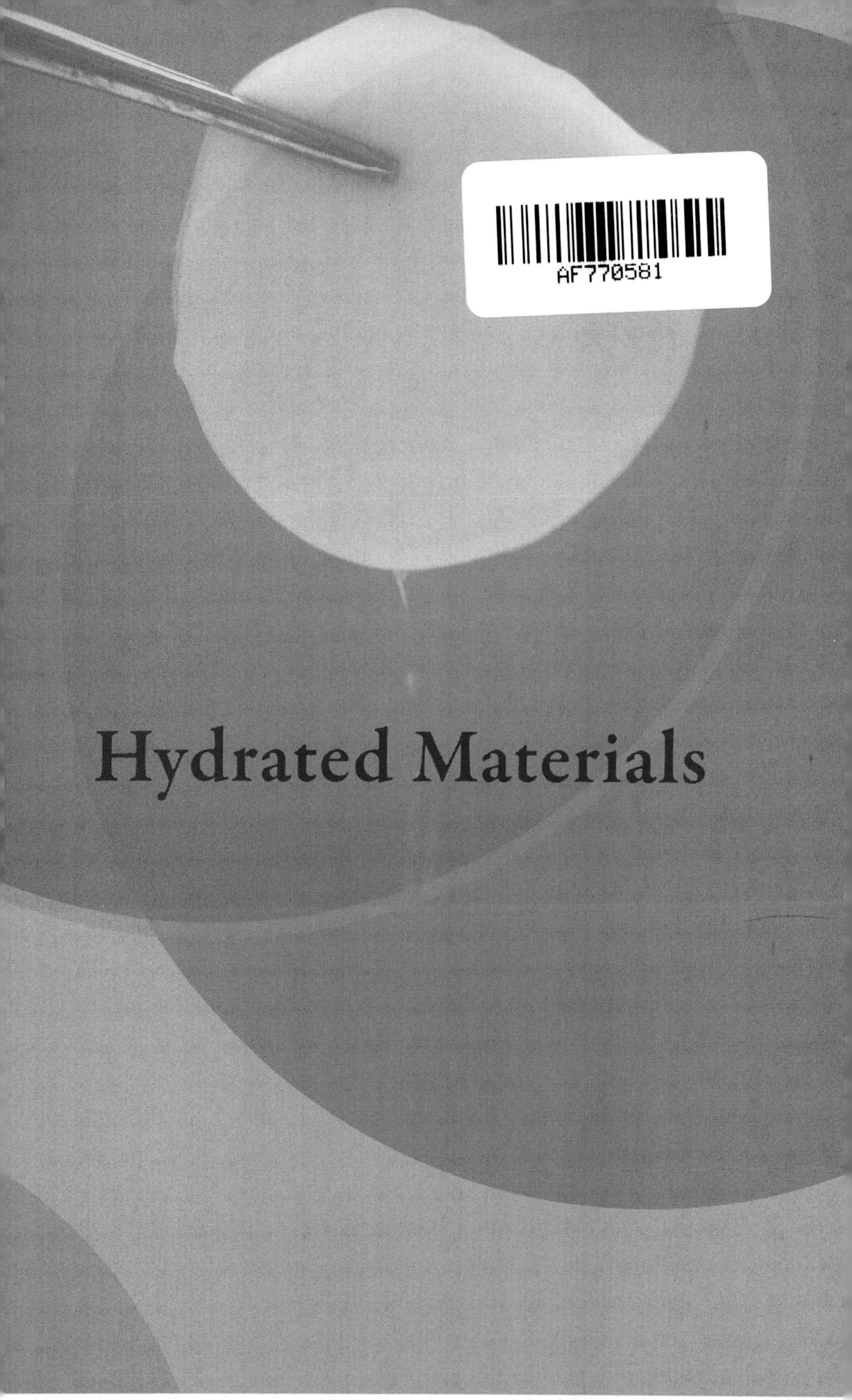

Hydrated Materials

Hydrated Materials

Applications in Biomedicine and the Environment

edited by

Yoshitaka Nakanishi

Pan Stanford Publishing

Published by

Pan Stanford Publishing Pte. Ltd.
Penthouse Level, Suntec Tower 3
8 Temasek Boulevard
Singapore 038988

Email: editorial@panstanford.com
Web: www.panstanford.com

British Library Cataloguing-in-Publication Data
A catalogue record for this book is available from the British Library.

Hydrated Materials: Applications in Biomedicine and the Environment

ISBN 978-981-4463-22-5 (Hardcover)
ISBN 978-981-4463-23-2 (eBook)

Printed in the USA

Contents

Preface

Water covers more than 70% of the earth's surface and is an essential and major component of all living matter. However, artificially hydrated materials, including hydrophilic materials, are far fewer than one might expect. Currently, these materials are in a state of development for applications in fields such as biomedicine, environmental engineering, and industrial engineering. So what do they hold for the future?

This book is a great introduction to hydrated materials for anyone unfamiliar with the topic. Readers can expect this book to be one of the first steps on the path to deepen the understanding of hydrated materials. Within this book they can expect to find academic and practical content, which will give them a feel of both theoretical and real- world problems; fundamental lectures, which will help them to develop a strong knowledge base; examples of latest issues, which will inform them of the direction of current research; hydrated materials defined in a simple manner and explanation for their effective use as a beginner; and a veritable cornucopia of practical examples in a range of fields, which can be employed to fully understand the topic.

I thank all chapter authors for their participation, cooperation, and patience, without which this book would not have been possible.

Yoshitaka Nakanishi
Spring 2015

Chapter 1

Mechanics of Materials

Mitsugu Todo
Research Institute for Applied Mechanics, Kyushu University, Japan
todo@riam.kyushu-u.ac.jp

1.1 Introduction

When an engineering material or a biological tissue is subjected to forces, it is deformed depending on its mechanical characteristics and the amount and direction of the forces. It is crucial to understand such mechanical response of the material from the standpoint of mechanical design when it is supposed to be used as a part of mechanical device. It is also fundamental to characterise the mechanical behaviour of the tissue from the biomechanical point of view because the remodelling of the tissue is known to be controlled by the mechanical environment surrounding the tissue and its mechanical properties. The macroscopic deformation behaviour of materials is usually characterised by expressing the relationship between the stress and the strain. Fundamental stress–strain relation can be obtained from mechanical tests such as tensile, compression and shear tests. Multi-axial mechanical tests are also sometimes performed to understand more complex mechanical

Hydrated Materials: Applications in Biomedicine and the Environment
Edited by Yoshitaka Nakanishi

ISBN 978-981-4463-22-5 (Hardcover), 978-981-4463-23-2 (eBook)
www.panstanford.com

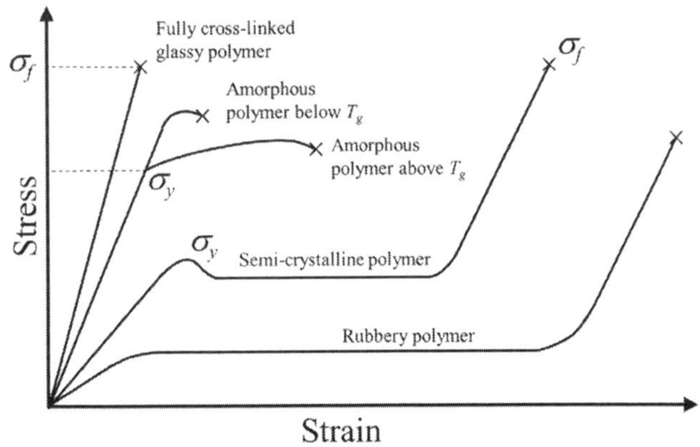

Figure 1.1 Stress–strain behaviour of various kinds of polymer.

response of the materials. The basic mechanical properties such as elastic moduli, Poisson's ratio, yield strength and failure strength are then determined from the testing results obtained. It is however very difficult to characterise the three-dimensional mechanical response of the materials, although in the most of real situations, they are subjected to three-dimensional loadings. As examples, the stress–strain relations of various types of polymers under tensile condition are shown in Fig. 1.1. These macroscopic mechanical characteristics strongly depend on the microstructures and the rheological conditions of macromolecules of the polymers.

The continuum mechanics approaches such as elasticity, viscoelasticity or plasticity have been utilised to theoretically characterise the stress–strain relations of materials and tissues. The elasticity is simply understood to be a mechanics that deals with totally reversible deformation, while the plasticity tries to express irreversible deformation with permanent strain mathematically. The viscoelasticity deals with time-dependent deformations such as creep and stress relaxation. Each of the mechanics theories can be used with equations and material parameters that differ from material to material. Those parameters are usually determined through mechanical tests experimentally.

In this chapter, the basic mathematical formulae appeared in each mechanics theories are described briefly.

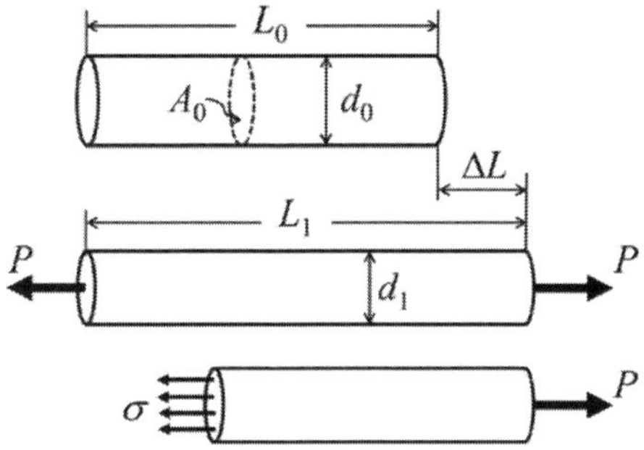

Figure 1.2 Cylindrical rod under tensile loading.

1.2 Strain

When a material is loaded, the change in the material's physical configuration can be described using a non-dimensional quantity called *strain*. Fundamentally, there are two types of strain: *normal strain* and *shear strain*. The normal strain is defined as the extension or compression in the direction of the applied load. As a simple example, we see a round bar subjected to a uniaxial load, as shown in Fig. 1.2. In this case, the strain in the axial direction is defined as:

$$\varepsilon = \frac{L_1 - L_0}{L_0} = \frac{\Delta L}{L_0} \tag{1.1}$$

It is also noted that the bar shrinks uniformly in the lateral direction, and the strain is defined as:

$$\varepsilon' = \frac{d_1 - d_0}{d_0} = \frac{\Delta d}{d_0} \tag{1.2}$$

The ratio of the strain in the lateral direction to the strain in the axial direction is known as *Poisson's ratio* and expressed by:

$$\nu = -\frac{\varepsilon'}{\varepsilon} \tag{1.3}$$

Poisson's ratio is known to be between 0 and 0.5.

A rectangular solid subjected to a shearing force slopes by the angle θ as shown in Fig. 1.3, and the shear strain is defined as:

$$\gamma = \frac{\Delta l}{l} = \tan\theta \approx \theta \tag{1.4}$$

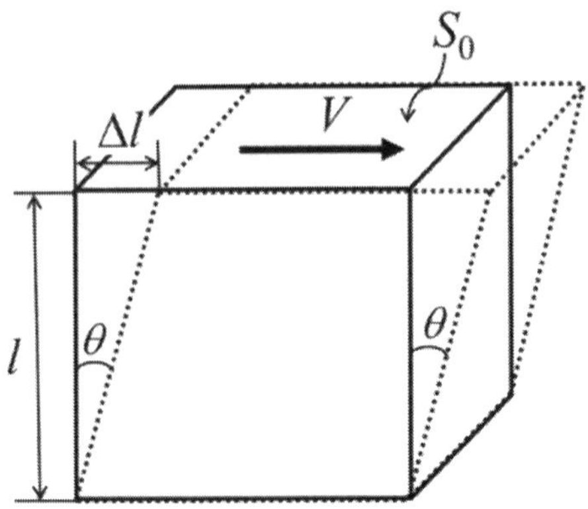

Figure 1.3 Rectangular solid under shear loading.

In general, if it is assumed that all strains are small, the components of normal strain are defined as follows:

$$\varepsilon_x = \frac{\partial u}{\partial x}, \quad \varepsilon_y = \frac{\partial v}{\partial y}, \quad \varepsilon_z = \frac{\partial w}{\partial z} \tag{1.5}$$

where u, v and w are the components of displacement in the x, y and z directions, respectively. Similarly, the components of shear strain are defined by:

$$\gamma_{xy} = \frac{\partial u}{\partial y} + \frac{\partial v}{\partial x}, \quad \gamma_{yz} = \frac{\partial v}{\partial z} + \frac{\partial w}{\partial y}, \quad \gamma_{zx} = \frac{\partial w}{\partial x} + \frac{\partial u}{\partial z} \tag{1.6}$$

1.3 Stress

Stress is understood as the transmission of force through deformable materials, and the force acting on the surface of unit area. For example, in a simple uniaxial loading case as shown in Fig. 1.2, *tensile stress* is defined as:

$$\sigma = \frac{P}{A_0} \tag{1.7}$$

Shear stress is also understood as the shearing force acting on the surface of unit area. Therefore, in the rectangular solid subjected to a shearing force V shown in Fig. 1.3, the shear stress is expressed as:

$$\tau = \frac{V}{S_0} \tag{1.8}$$

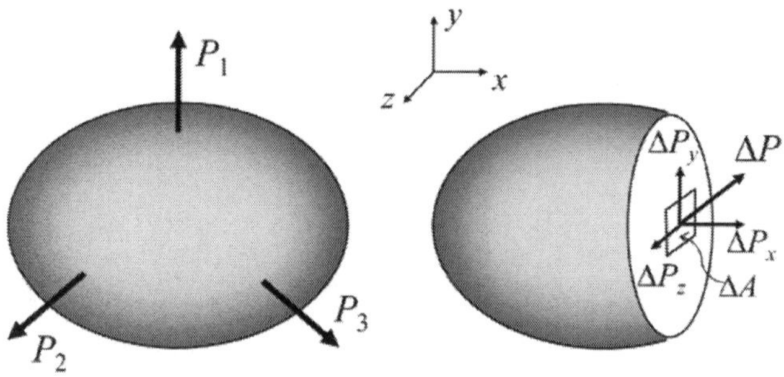

Figure 1.4 An arbitrary solid under three-dimensional loading condition.

We consider a body subjected to a force vector $\boldsymbol{P}$ having the rectangular components P_1, P_2 and P_3 as shown in Fig. 1.4. In a certain cross-sectional area perpendicular to the x-axis, the force vector $\Delta\boldsymbol{P}$ acting on the surface can be decomposed of three components ΔP_x, ΔP_y and ΔP_z. Stress components are then defined as follows:

$$\sigma_x = \lim_{\Delta A \to 0} \frac{\Delta P_x}{\Delta A}, \qquad \tau_{xy} = \lim_{\Delta A \to 0} \frac{\Delta P_y}{\Delta A}, \qquad \tau_{xz} = \lim_{\Delta A \to 0} \frac{\Delta P_z}{\Delta A} \tag{1.9}$$

In a more general way, an infinitesimally small cube inside of the solid, as shown in Fig. 1.4, is often considered to express stress tensor as illustrated in Fig. 1.5. In this configuration, there are three normal stresses and six shear stresses existing on the surfaces. The

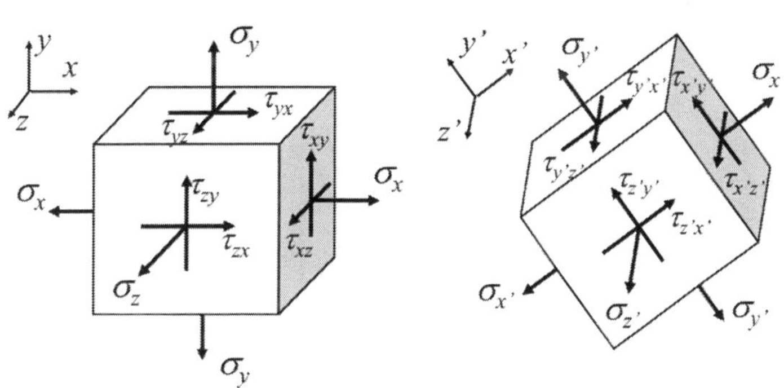

Figure 1.5 Stress components acting on the surfaces of a small cube.

stress tensor is defined by:

$$\sigma = \begin{bmatrix} \sigma_x & \tau_{xy} & \tau_{xz} \\ \tau_{yx} & \sigma_y & \tau_{yz} \\ \tau_{zx} & \tau_{zy} & \sigma_z \end{bmatrix} \tag{1.10}$$

It can be proved from the theory of elasticity that this tensor must be symmetric, that is, $\tau_{ij} = \tau_{ji}$. Therefore, the stress tensor actually has three shear components. If the cube is rotated as shown in Fig. 1.5, the stresses in the new position will be related to the original stresses, but they will generally not be the same. The stress components in the original rectangular Cartesian coordinate system x, y, z are expressed by σ_{ij} where $i = 1$, 2 or 3 and $j = 1$, 2 or 3, corresponding to x, y and z, respectively. Similarly, the stress components in the new coordinate system x', y', z' are denoted by σ'_{km} where $k = 1$, 2 or 3 and $m = 1$, 2 or 3, corresponding to x', y' and z', respectively. Then, the stress components are transformed according to the tensor transformation law:

$$\sigma'_{km} = \sigma_{ji}\alpha_{kj}\alpha_{mi} \tag{1.11}$$

where α_{ki} denotes the direction cosine of the x'_k axis ($x'_1 = x'$, $x'_2 = y'$, $x'_3 = z'$) with respect to the x_i axis ($x_1 = x$, $x_2 = y$, $x_3 = z$). In these formulae, the summation convention of the index is used.

At every point in a solid, there exists a plane, called a principal plane, where only the normal stress is acting on the plane and there is no shear stress acting on that surface. These normal stresses are called *principal stresses* and usually denoted by σ_1, σ_2 and σ_3 in three-dimensional stress states.

1.4 Constitutive Equations

The mechanical responses of materials are characterised by the relationships between stress and strain from the continuum mechanics point of view. These theoretical descriptions are called *constitutive equations*. A wide variety of materials from soft polymer to hard ceramics exist. Therefore, many constitutive equations describing such variety of materials must be developed.

1.4.1 *Linear Elasticity*

The simplest formula is the constitutive equation for the linear elastic material under uniaxial tensile loading as shown in Fig. 1.2. In this case, stress is proportional to strain and the stress–strain relation is called *Hooke's Law* and given by:

$$\sigma = E\varepsilon \tag{1.12}$$

where E is called *Young's modulus*. Similarly, the linear relation of shear stress and shear strain is expressed as:

$$\tau = G\gamma \tag{1.13}$$

Where G is called *shear modulus*, and can be written as a function of E and ν as follows:

$$G = \frac{E}{2\left(1+\nu\right)} \tag{1.14}$$

Hooke's Law can be extended to a multi-axial loading condition. The principle of linear superposition is utilised to obtain the generalised Hooke's Law for a three-dimensional stress state as follows:

$$\varepsilon_x = \frac{1}{E}\left[\sigma_x - \nu\left(\sigma_y + \sigma_z\right)\right] \tag{1.15a}$$

$$\varepsilon_y = \frac{1}{E}\left[\sigma_y - \nu\left(\sigma_z + \sigma_x\right)\right] \tag{1.15b}$$

$$\varepsilon_z = \frac{1}{E}\left[\sigma_z - \nu\left(\sigma_x + \sigma_y\right)\right] \tag{1.15c}$$

$$\gamma_{xy} = \frac{\tau_{xy}}{G}, \quad \gamma_{yz} = \frac{\tau_{yz}}{G}, \quad \gamma_{zx} = \frac{\tau_{zx}}{G} \tag{1.15d}$$

Equation (1.15) can also be written by the tensor form:

$$\varepsilon_{ij} = \frac{1+\nu}{E}\sigma_{ij} - \frac{\nu}{E}\delta_{ij}\sigma_{kk} \tag{1.16}$$

where δ_{ij} is the Kronecker delta, which has the value 1 if $i = j$, and zero if $i \neq j$

1.4.2 *Viscoelasticity*

When a body is suddenly strained and then the strain is maintained constant, the corresponding stresses decrease with time. This mechanical phenomenon is call *stress relaxation*. On the contrary, if the body is suddenly stressed and then the stress is maintained constant, the body continues to deform. This phenomenon is called *creep*. If the body is subjected to a cyclic loading, the stress–strain relationship in the loading process is usually somewhat different from that in the unloading process, and the phenomenon is called *hysteresis*. The features of hysteresis, stress relaxation and creep are found in many natural and engineering materials, and such mechanical behaviours are theoretically characterised by *viscoelasticity*.

Mechanical models have been developed to discuss the viscoelastic behaviour of materials. Three representative mechanical models for simplified viscoelastic behaviour are shown in Fig. 1.6, and they are called the *Maxwell model*, the *Voigt model* and the *Kelvin model*, respectively, all of which are composed of combinations of linear springs with spring constant E and dashpots with coefficient of viscosity η. A linear spring is supposed to produce instantaneously a deformation proportional to the load and therefore, the strain ε of

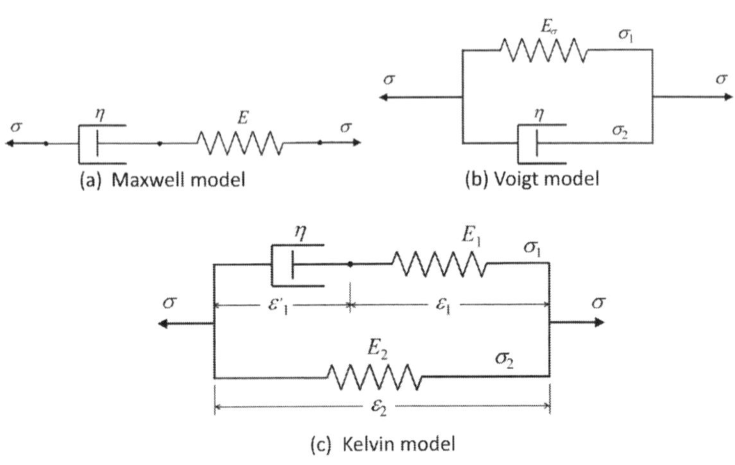

Figure 1.6 Three fundamental viscoelastic models.

the spring is related to σ by Hook's Law Eq. (1.12), that is, $\sigma = E\varepsilon$. A dashpot is supposed to produce a velocity proportional to the load at any instance and therefore, the velocity of deflection $d\varepsilon/dt$ in the dashpot is related to σ by $\sigma = \eta d\varepsilon/dt$. The total velocity in the Maxwell model is then given by the sum of the contributions from the spring and the dashpot such that:

$$\frac{d\varepsilon}{dt} = \frac{1}{E}\frac{d\sigma}{dt} + \frac{\sigma}{\eta} \tag{1.17}$$

For the Voigt model, the spring and the dashpot have the same strain. The total stress σ is therefore

$$\sigma = \sigma_1 + \sigma_2 = E\varepsilon + \eta\frac{d\varepsilon}{dt} \tag{1.18}$$

For the Kelvin model, the strain ε is decomposed of ε_1 of the spring and ε_1' of the dashpot. The total stress σ is the sum of the stress σ_1 from the Maxwell element and the stress σ_2 from the single spring. Thus, the following equations are obtained:

$$\varepsilon = \varepsilon_1 + \varepsilon_1' \quad \sigma = \sigma_1 + \sigma_2 \tag{1.19}$$

and

$$\sigma_1 = E_1\varepsilon_1 = \eta\frac{d\varepsilon_1}{dt} \quad \sigma_2 = E_2\varepsilon_2 \tag{1.20}$$

By combining these equations, the relationship between the stress and the strain is given by:

$$\sigma + \frac{\eta}{E_1}\frac{d\sigma}{dt} = \eta\left(1 + \frac{E_2}{E_1}\right)\frac{d\varepsilon}{dt} + E_2\varepsilon \tag{1.21}$$

This equation is also expressed as:

$$\sigma + \tau_\varepsilon\frac{d\sigma}{dt} = E_R\left(\varepsilon + \tau_\sigma\frac{d\varepsilon}{dt}\right) \tag{1.22}$$

where

$$\tau_\varepsilon = \frac{\eta}{E_1}, \quad \tau_\sigma = \frac{\eta}{E_2}\left(1 + \frac{E_2}{E_1}\right), \quad E_R = E_2 \tag{1.23}$$

The constant τ_ε is called the relaxation time for constant strain, whereas τ_σ is called the relaxation time for constant stress.

In order to understand the fundamental mechanical responses of these three models, we introduce a unit-step function $U(t)$ defined as:

$$U(t) = \begin{cases} 1 & : \quad t > 0 \\ \dfrac{1}{2} & : \quad t = 0 \\ 0 & : \quad t < 0 \end{cases} \tag{1.24}$$

By solving these equations for $\varepsilon(t)$ when $\sigma(t)$ is the unit-step function $U(t)$, we obtain:

From Maxwell model

$$D_c(t) = \left(\frac{1}{E} + \frac{1}{\eta}t\right) U(t) \tag{1.25}$$

From Voigt model

$$D_c(t) = \frac{1}{E}\left(1 - e^{-Et/\eta}\right) U(t) \tag{1.26}$$

From Kelvin model

$$D_c(t) = \frac{1}{E_R}\left[1 - \left(1 - \frac{\tau_\varepsilon}{\tau_\sigma}\right) e^{-t/\tau_\sigma}\right] U(t) \tag{1.27}$$

These $D_c(t)$ are called *creep compliance*. On the contrary, by solving the equations for $\sigma(t)$ when $\varepsilon(t)$ is $U(t)$, we obtain:

From Maxwell model

$$E_r(t) = Ee^{-Et/\eta}U(t) \tag{1.28}$$

From Voigt model

$$E_r(t) = \eta\delta(t) + E\,U(t) \tag{1.29}$$

From Kelvin model

$$E_r(t) = E_R\left[1 - \left(1 - \frac{\tau_\sigma}{\tau_\varepsilon}\right) e^{-t/\tau_\varepsilon}\right] U(t) \tag{1.30}$$

These $E_r(t)$ are called *relaxation modulus*. The $\delta(t)$ is called Dirac-delta function and defined by:

$$\delta(t) = 0 \quad : \quad t < 0 \text{ and } t > 0 \tag{1.31a}$$

$$\int_{-\varepsilon}^{\varepsilon} f(t)\,\delta(t)\,dt = f(0) \quad : \quad \varepsilon > 0 \tag{1.31b}$$

where $f(t)$ is an arbitrary function, continuous at $t = 0$. These $D_c(t)$ and $E_r(t)$ are illustrated in Figs. 1.7 and 1.8, respectively.

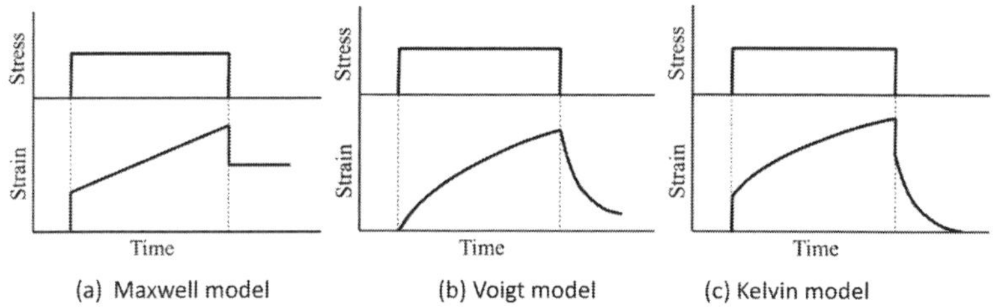

Figure 1.7 Creep compliances of three models.

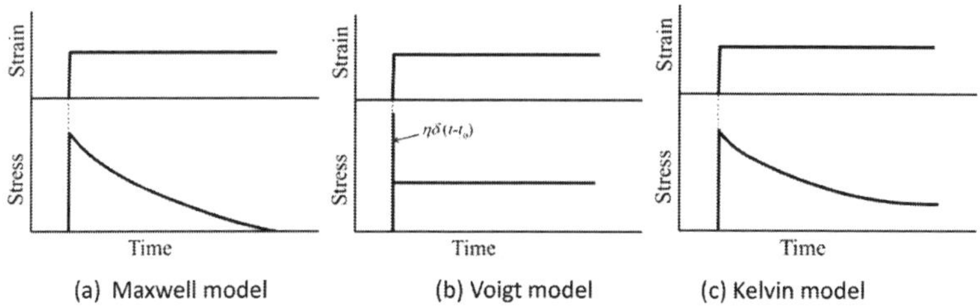

Figure 1.8 Relaxation moduli of three models.

More generalised models can be developed to express the viscoelastic responses of materials. Typical examples of such models are the generalised Maxwell model and the generalised Voigt model (also called generalised Kelvin model) that are constructed as a series of the unit models as shown in Figs. 1.9 and 1.10. For the generalised Maxwell model shown in Fig. 1.9, the stress–strain relation is expressed as:

$$\sigma(t) = \left[E_e + \sum_i \frac{E_i}{(D + 1/\tau_i)} D \right] \varepsilon(t) \tag{1.32}$$

where $D = d/dt$ and $\tau_i = \eta_i / E_i$. For the generalised Voigt model shown in Fig. 1.10, the stress–strain relation is given by:

$$\varepsilon(t) = \left[C_e + \sum_i \frac{C_i}{\tau_i (D + 1/\tau_i)} D \right] \sigma(t) \tag{1.33}$$

where

$$C_e = \frac{1}{E_e}, \quad C_i = \frac{1}{E_i}, \quad \tau_i = \frac{\eta_i}{E_i} \tag{1.34}$$

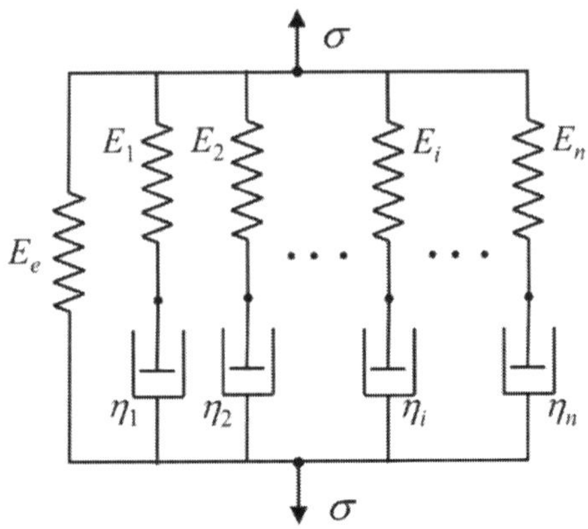

Figure 1.9 Generalised Maxwell model.

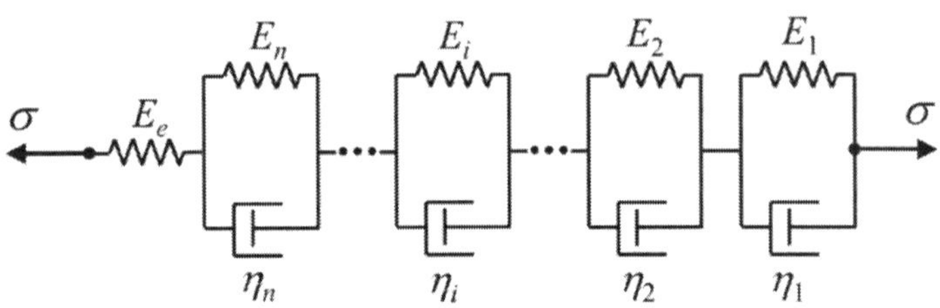

Figure 1.10 Generalised Voigt (Kelvin) model.

1.5 Elastoplasticity

Most of engineering metals and plastics exhibit irreversible non-linear deformation when these materials are loaded beyond their elastic limits. Such deformation is called plastic deformation. It should be noted that the final state of deformation depends not only on the final loading but also on the loading history. To express such elastic–plastic deformation theoretically, yield criteria, that define the transition point from reversible elastic to irreversible plastic deformation, need to be developed. Furthermore, the incremental theory (the flow theory) and the total strain theory (or the deformation theory) has been established to describe the plastic deformation mathematically.

Some idealised stress–strain relations have been introduced in order to express the elastic–plastic stress–strain behaviour mathematically. These stress–strain relations are schematically illustrated in Fig. 1.11. It is mathematically convenient to decompose the elastoplastic stress–strain behaviour into the linear elastic deformation region and the subsequent plastic deformation region. The plastic stress–strain behaviour can be expressed by both linear and nonlinear functions. In the perfectly plastic deformation, the stress keeps constant value equivalent to the yield strength in the plastic region [Fig. 1.11(a)]. The linear and nonlinear work-hardenings exhibit linear and nonlinear increasing behaviours of stress with increasing strain in the plastic region as shown in Fig. 1.11(b and c), respectively. For a mathematical simplicity, exponential function is sometimes introduced to express the nonlinear work-hardening behaviour as shown in Fig. 1.11(d).

1.5.1 *Yield Criteria*

The strain ε_{ij} in an elastic–plastic material is decomposed of the elastic and plastic contributions such that

$$\varepsilon_{ij} = \varepsilon_{ij}^{e} + \varepsilon_{ij}^{p} \tag{1.35}$$

where ε_{ij}^{e} and ε_{ij}^{p} denote the elastic and plastic contributions, respectively. The elastic component is related to the stress σ_{ij} by the generalised Hooke's Law:

$$\sigma_{ij} = C_{ijkl}\varepsilon_{kl} \tag{1.36}$$

where C_{ijkl} is the tensor of elastic constants. Symmetry of the stress and strain tensors requires that $C_{ijkl} = C_{jikl}$ and $C_{ijkl} = C_{ijlk}$, respectively. If the stress level is lower than the yielding point, then the plastic strain component is identically zero. When yielding takes place, the plastic deformation is assumed to be incompressible, that is:

$$\varepsilon_{ii}^{p} = 0 \tag{1.37}$$

A yield criterion is required to assess whether or not plastic deformation has occurred. It is assumed that a yield function exists such that:

$$f = f(\sigma_{ij}) \tag{1.38}$$

This is a function of the current state of stress σ_{ij}. The yield surface $f = 0$ represents a hypersurface in the nine-dimensional Euclidean

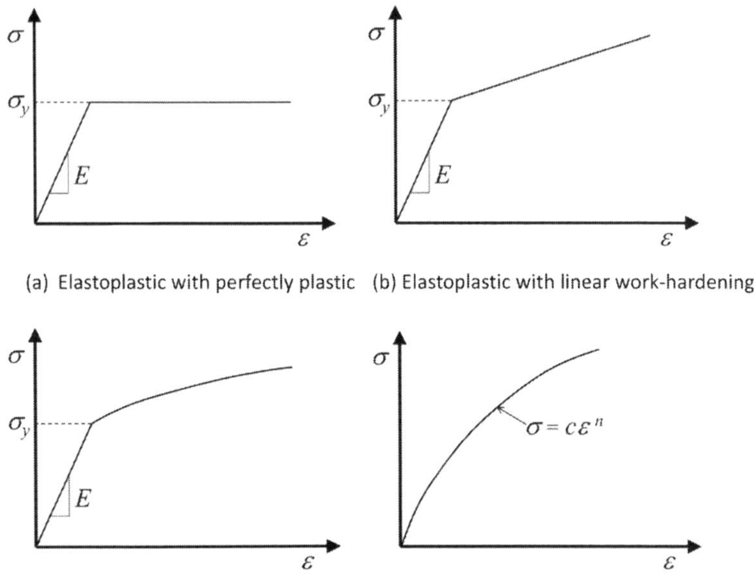

(a) Elastoplastic with perfectly plastic (b) Elastoplastic with linear work-hardening

(c) Elastoplastic with nonlinear work-hardening (d) Parabolic work-hardening

Figure 1.11 Idealised elastic–plastic stress–strain relations.

space σ_{ij}. In general, the yield surface can expand (isotropic hardening), translate (kinematic hardening) or both during plastic deformation. All current stress must lie either on or inside ($f \leq 0$) this surface, but never outside ($f > 0$) it. All stress states within the surface are elastic whereas during plastic deformation the current stress state must be on the yield surface.

For isotropic material behaviour, the yield function must be an isotropic function of the stress. This requires that:

$$f = f(I_1, I_2, I_3) \tag{1.39}$$

where I_i are the stress invariants defined by:

$$I_1 = \sigma_x + \sigma_y + \sigma_z \tag{1.40a}$$

$$I_2 = (\sigma_x\sigma_y + \sigma_y\sigma_z + \sigma_z\sigma_x) - \tau_{xy}^2 - \tau_{yz}^2 - \tau_{zx}^2 \tag{1.40b}$$

$$I_2 = \begin{vmatrix} \sigma_x & \tau_{xy} & \tau_{zx} \\ \tau_{xy} & \sigma_y & \tau_{yz} \\ \tau_{zx} & \tau_{yz} & \sigma_z \end{vmatrix} \tag{1.40c}$$

Since these invariants can be expressed in terms of the principal stresses, then alternatively:

$$f = f(\sigma_1, \sigma_2, \sigma_3) \tag{1.41}$$

Yielding of most metals is not influenced by a moderate hydrostatic pressure:

$$p = (\sigma_x + \sigma_y + \sigma_z)/3 = I_1/3 \tag{1.42}$$

For such cases, the yield function is independent of I_1 and depends only on the deviatoric stresses s_{ij} which is defined by:

$$s_{ij} = \sigma_{ij} - \frac{1}{3}\delta_{ij}\sigma_{ii} \tag{1.43}$$

Therefore, for isotropic behaviour:

$$f = f(J_2, J_3) \tag{1.44}$$

where J_2 and J_3 are the second and the third invariants of the deviatoric stress tensor, respectively, and given by:

$$J_2 = \frac{1}{2}s_{ij}s_{ij} \quad J_3 = \frac{1}{3}s_{ij}s_{ik}s_{jk} \tag{1.45}$$

The von Mises and the Tresca yield conditions are widely used as yield criteria in the material engineering field. The von Mises yield function is expressed as:

$$f = J_2 - k^2 \tag{1.46}$$

where the parameter k depends on the strain history for a work hardening material and assumes a constant for a perfectly plastic material. In terms of the principal stresses, the von Mises yield surface is defined by:

$$f = \frac{1}{6}\left[(\sigma_1 - \sigma_2)^2 + (\sigma_2 - \sigma_3)^2 + (\sigma_3 - \sigma_1)^2\right] - k^2 = 0 \tag{1.47}$$

If we introduce a condition of pure shear with $\sigma_1 = -\sigma_3 = \sigma$ and $\sigma_2 = 0$ where τ is the yield stress in shear, then Eq. (1.45) results in:

$$k = \tau \tag{1.48}$$

On the other hand, if we introduce a condition of uniaxial tension with $\sigma_1 = \sigma_y$ and $\sigma_2 = \sigma_3 = 0$ where σ_y is the yield stress in uniaxial tension, then:

$$k = \frac{\sigma_y}{\sqrt{3}} \tag{1.49}$$

This result implies that the parameter k can be determined from uniaxial tensile test. The von Mises yield surface is a circular cylindrical surface whose axis is the ray $\sigma_1 = \sigma_2 = \sigma_3$

The Tresca criterion was derived from the assumption that yielding occurs when the maximum shear stress in the material reaches the yield stress k in shear. Therefore, the Tresca criterion can be expressed using the principal stresses such that:

$$\max\left[|\sigma_1 - \sigma_2|, |\sigma_2 - \sigma_3|, |\sigma_3 - \sigma_1|\right] = 2k \qquad (1.50)$$

The Tresca yield surface is a regular hexagonal cylinder with the axis $\sigma_1 = \sigma_2 = \sigma_3$ in the principal stress space.

1.5.2 *Incremental Plasticity*

From Eq. (1.35), strain increment may be expressed as:

$$d\varepsilon_{ij} = d\varepsilon_{ij}^{e} + d\varepsilon_{ij}^{p} \qquad (1.51)$$

From Eq. (1.15), the elastic strain increment $d\varepsilon_{ij}^{e}$ is given by:

$$d\varepsilon_{ij}^{e} = \frac{1+\nu}{E} d\sigma_{ij} - \frac{\nu}{E}\delta_{ij} d\sigma_{kk} \qquad (1.52)$$

By introducing von Mises yield criterion, the plastic strain increment $d\varepsilon_{ij}^{p}$ is expressed as:

$$d\varepsilon_{ij}^{p} = \frac{3}{2}\frac{s_{ij}}{\bar{\sigma}}\frac{}{H'} d\bar{\sigma} \qquad (1.53)$$

where s_{ij} is the deviatoric stress defined by Eq. (1.43), and $\bar{\sigma}$ is the effective stress which is defined by:

$$\bar{\sigma} = (3J_2)^{1/2} = \left(\frac{3}{2}s_{ij}s_{ij}\right)^{1/2} \qquad (1.54)$$

The corresponding effective strain is defined by:

$$\bar{\varepsilon}^{p} = \left(\frac{2}{3}\varepsilon_{ij}^{p}\varepsilon_{ij}^{p}\right)^{1/2} \qquad (1.55)$$

Therefore, the effective stress and strain increments are expressed as:

$$d\bar{\sigma} = \left(\frac{3}{2}ds_{ij}ds_{ij}\right)^{1/2} \qquad (1.56a)$$

$$d\bar{\varepsilon}^{p} = \left(\frac{2}{3}d\varepsilon_{ij}^{p}d\varepsilon_{ij}^{p}\right)^{1/2} \qquad (1.56b)$$

H' is the slope of the equivalent stress—the equivalent plastic strain curve at the current effective stress. Substitution of Eqs. (1.52) and

(1.53) into Eq. (1.51) yields:

$$d\varepsilon_{ij} = \frac{1+\nu}{E} d\sigma_{ij} - \frac{\nu}{E}\delta_{ij} d\sigma_{kk} + \frac{3}{2}\frac{s_{ij}}{\bar{\sigma}}\frac{1}{H'} d\bar{\sigma} \tag{1.57}$$

1.5.3 *Deformation Plasticity*

The deformation theory of plasticity is actually a nonlinear elasticity theory and therefore has very definite limitations. Nevertheless, it offers certain mathematical simplifications that make its useful. In the deformation theory, it is assumed that:

$$\varepsilon_{ij}^{p} = \phi\, s_{ij} \tag{1.58}$$

where ϕ is a scalar function of the stress invariants and plastic strains. From Eqs. (1.53) and (1.58), one obtains:

$$\phi = \frac{3}{2}\frac{\bar{\varepsilon}^{p}}{\bar{\sigma}} \tag{1.59}$$

Substitution of Eqs. (1.15), (1.58) and (1.59) into Eq. (1.35) yields:

$$\varepsilon_{ij} = \frac{1+\nu}{E}\sigma_{ij} - \frac{\nu}{E}\delta_{ij}\sigma_{kk} + \frac{3}{2}\frac{\bar{\varepsilon}^{p}}{\bar{\sigma}} s_{ij} \tag{1.60}$$

The principal limitation of the deformation theory of plasticity is reflected by Eq. (1.58). The plastic strains depend only on the current state of stress and are independent of the path leading to this state.

Bibliography

1. Gere JM, Timoshenko SP (1984) *Mechanics of Materials*, 2nd ed, PWS Engineering, Boston, MA.
2. Kanninen MF, Popelar CH (1985) *Advanced Fracture Mechanics*, Oxford University Press, New York, NY.
3. Fung YC (1993) *Biomechanics: Mechanical Properties of Living Tissues*, 2nd ed, Springer-Verlag, New York, NY.
4. Meyers MA, Chawla KK (2009) *Mechanical Behavior of Materials*, 2nd ed, Cambridge University Press, UK.
5. Pruitt LA, Chakravartula AM (2011) *Mechanics of Biomaterials: Fundamental Principles for Implant Design*, Cambridge University Press, UK.

Chapter 2

Tribology: Friction, Wear and Lubrication

Kazuyuki Yagi
Department of Mechanical Engineering, Kyushu University, 744 Motooka, Fukuoka-city, Fukuoka 819-0395, Japan
yagik@mech.kyushu-u.ac.jp

This chapter describes the fundamental of tribology. Tribology is the science and engineering of interacting surfaces with relative motion. Interacting areas can be found in machinery as well as human body. In some contacting areas, low friction and wear are desirable for requirements of high efficient and safe operation. Lubrication is conducted to decrease friction and wear. On the other hand, there also exist contacting areas in which high friction and wear are required such as clutches, tires and erasers. It is important for tribological engineers and scientists to control and use effectively functions obtained from interacting surfaces such as friction, wear and lubrication. In this chapter, the principles of friction, wear and lubrication are introduced.

2.1 Introduction of Tribology

The term 'tribology' is defined as the science and engineering of interacting surfaces in relative motion in 1966 by a committee

Hydrated Materials: Applications in Biomedicine and the Environment
Edited by Yoshitaka Nakanishi

ISBN 978-981-4463-22-5 (Hardcover), 978-981-4463-23-2 (eBook)
www.panstanford.com

of the Organization for Economic Cooperation and Development. Interacting surfaces can be found everywhere. Vehicles have contacting areas between the ground and tires at which traction force is generated for movement. Pencils and erasers work by making a contact area between a pencil and a paper. Machines have many frictional and lubricated areas formed by contacting surfaces. Human body also has many interacting surfaces in human joints. Frictional areas have many complex and important phenomena related to mechanics, physics, material science and chemistry, which were attractive for scientists as well as engineers.

Friction is most accessible phenomenon for human, which is resistance force against movement under normal loading and is energy dissipation process. Normally, frictional force should be reduced for frictional areas. However, human being cannot walk and catch anything by hands unless frictional force takes place. Wear is material waste process of surfaces during frictional movement. As wear occurs in frictional area, debris particles are generated as a result of detachment parts of the surfaces, which cause further damage of frictional surfaces. The function of lubrication is to support normal load by thin film to prevent from direct contacts of mating surfaces and to decrease friction and wear. Liquid lubricant is usually used to achieve the formation of a fluid film in which viscous flow occurs. However, gas and a few atomic layers adsorbed on surfaces also posses the function of 'lubrication'.

The goal of 'tribology' is to control and use effectively friction, wear and lubrication depending on requirements. For rolling bearings used in spindles and shafts, safe and long-time operation with low frictional force and wear is required, while clutches equipped in transmissions and tires need high frictional force to transfer high power. The impact of reduction of friction and wear is not small for the economical aspect as well as engineering one. The reduction of frictional force of each rolling bearing and gear may be small. However, many rolling bearings and gears are used in one machine. The accumulation of the frictional reduction becomes a great impact on energy savings. If the longer life operation is achieved as a result of overcoming tribological problems, no exchange of parts of machinery during short period become to be required.

2.2 Friction

Friction is a process of energy dissipation during sliding motion under normal loading. Friction is generated in the opposite direction of the sliding motion as a resistance force. Leonardo da Vinci found two laws of friction, which were again discovered and further developed by Guilaume Amontons and Caharles-Augustin de Coulomb. Four empirical laws are as follows:

- Frictional force is proportional to normal load.
- Frictional force is independent of apparent contact area.
- Frictional force is independent of sliding speed.
- The static frictional force is greater than the dynamic frictional force.

Amonton and Coulomb believed that the origin of friction would cause when one surface having roughness climbs another roughened surface. This hypothesis had well been recognised for more than five hundred years since Amonton thought. However, in accordance with progress of technology, it was found that frictional force increased when surfaces with small roughness were used [1]. Bowden and Tabor [2] suggested that friction would be generated by adhesive force when contacting asperities on the mating surfaces were detached.

Figure 2.1 shows the schematic of mating asperities under applied load. The real contact area between the asperities can be expressed when plastic deformation of the asperities occurs.

$$A_{\mathrm{r}} = \frac{W}{p_{\mathrm{m}}} \tag{2.1}$$

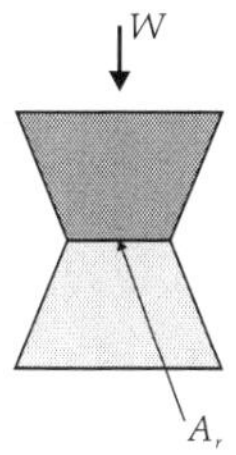

Figure 2.1 Adhesive force at asperity-asperity contact area.

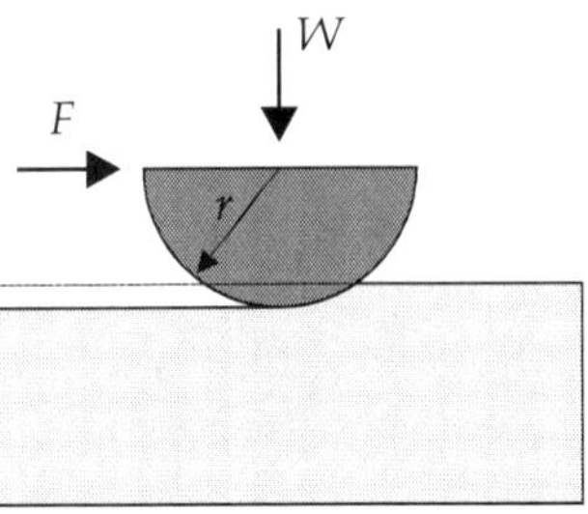

Figure 2.2 Ploughing force during sliding.

where A_r is the real contact area, W is the load and p_m is the hardness of softer asperity. Friction F_a and friction coefficient μ can be expressed as the following equation:

$$F_a = \left(\frac{W}{p_m}\right) s \qquad (2.2)$$

$$\mu = \frac{s}{p_m} \qquad (2.3)$$

where s is the shear stress by adhesive force. When load increases, the real contact area also increases proportionally. Therefore, the friction coefficient is constant. The hypothesis of adhesive force can explain three of the four empirical laws.

In the case where one surface is considerably softer than the other surface, ploughing action contributes to friction. Figure 2.2 shows the schematic of ploughing action.

When the asperity of harder material penetrated into softer surface to slide in the tangential direction, it is necessary to remove softer material during sliding. Friction by ploughing surface F_p can be expressed as follows.

$$F_p = A_p p_m \qquad (2.4)$$

where A_p is the reflected area to the sliding direction. The contribution of frictional force by ploughing action depends on the difference in hardness between the surfaces and geometrical shape. At least in metal–metal contacts, the influence of ploughing action on frictional force can be negligible.

As expressed Eq. (2.1), the real contact area is created as a result of plastic deformation by normal load under a static contact.

As sliding motion is added to normal load, frictional force also contributes to increase the real contact area. The mechanism of the increase in real contact area by frictional force is called 'junction growth'. The mechanism of junction growth can be explained by the following Von Mieses yield criterion:

$$p^2 + C\tau^2 = p_y^2 = Cs_{\mathrm{m}}^2 \tag{2.5}$$

where p is the normal stress, τ is the shear stress, p_y is the plastic flow stress under only normal load, s_{m} is the shear strength and C is an arbitrary constant. The value of C ranges from 3 to 25 [2]. The stresses p and p_y can be expressed as follows:

$$p = \frac{W}{A_{\mathrm{r}}} \tag{2.6}$$

$$\tau = \frac{F}{A_{\mathrm{r}}} \tag{2.7}$$

$$p_0 = \frac{W}{A_{\mathrm{r0}}} \tag{2.8}$$

where F is the frictional force, W is the normal force, A_{r} is the real contact area under normal and tangential forces and A_{r0} is the real contact area with only normal force W.

Substituting and rearranging gives:

$$\frac{A_{\mathrm{r}}}{A_{\mathrm{r0}}} = \frac{W/p}{W/p_{\mathrm{m}}} = \sqrt{1 + \alpha\left(\frac{F}{W}\right)^2} = \frac{1}{\sqrt{1 - (s/s_{\mathrm{m}})^2}} \tag{2.9}$$

$$\varphi = \frac{F}{W} = \frac{sA}{pA} = \frac{s}{p} = \frac{1}{\sqrt{\alpha\left((s/s_{\mathrm{m}})^2 - 1\right)}} \tag{2.10}$$

The above equations indicate that the real contact area increases to infinity as the shear force reach the shear strength of material s_{m}. as shown in Fig. 2.3. Actually, the surface starts to slide before the shear force s reaches s_{m} [3]. Consider a thin film with the shear strength s_{f} on the surface.

$$s_{\mathrm{f}} = ks_{\mathrm{m}} \tag{2.11}$$

Substituting the shear strength of the thin film s_{f} into Eq. (2.10) gives:

$$\frac{A}{A_0} = \frac{1}{\sqrt{1 - k^2}} \tag{2.12}$$

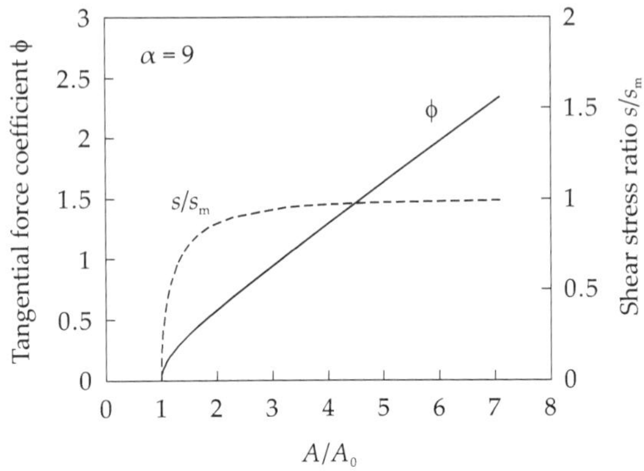

Figure 2.3 Increase of real contact area by frictional force.

$$\phi = \frac{k}{\sqrt{C\,(1-k^2)}} \tag{2.13}$$

Figure 2.4 shows the real contact area ratio A/A_0 and tangential friction coefficient ϕ for various shear strength ratios s_f/s_m. The values of A/A_0 and ϕ are significantly reduced as s_f/s_m decreases. According to the above equations, the combination between a thin

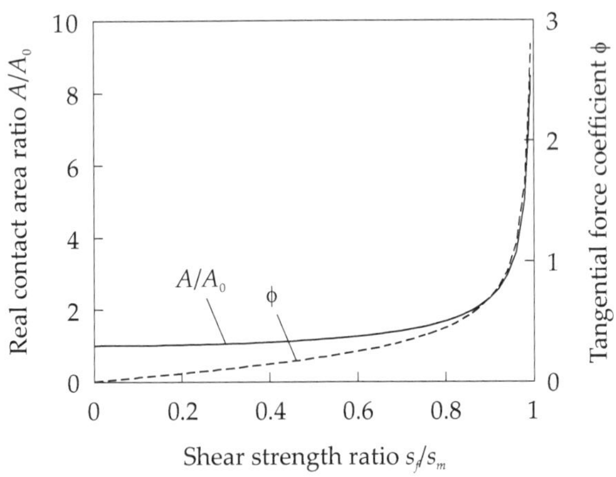

Figure 2.4 Real contact area ratio and tangential friction coefficient for various shear strength ratios.

film with low shear strength and a surface with high hardness is the best way to reduce the friction coefficient.

2.3 Wear

Wear is material waste at the interfaces between contacting bodies by friction during sliding. As wear occurs, wear debris particles are generated and then surface topography is changed. The occurrence of wear reduces efficiency and reliability of machinery to cause further damages of surfaces. On the other hand, there are also many techniques such as cutting, polishing, superfinishing, chemical and mechanical polishing (CMP) and running-in to utilise the wear phenomenon. The wear phenomenon is complex and is related to mechanical, physical and chemical mechanisms. To date, many investigations on wear have been conducted. However, no systematic way to predict and estimate quantitatively wear has been found.

The mode of wear can be classified into the following mechanisms:

- adhesive wear
- abrasive wear
- corrosive wear
- erosive wear

Adhesive wear occurs at real contact areas of contacting asperities because adhesive force detaches parts of the surfaces. Archard [4] explained the wear volume by adhesive wear using a simple model schematically shown in Fig. 2.1. It is assumed that there are the sum of real contact areas A_r composed of n of circular contacting points with radius a. As the upper asperity slides, the contact area decreases to reach 0. When the contact area equal to 0, another pair of asperities are assumed to start to contact. The number of contacts of asperities N during sliding in distance L can be expressed as follows:

$$N = \frac{nL}{2a} \tag{2.14}$$

Substituting $W = p_{\mathrm{m}} A_{\mathrm{r}}$ and $A_{\mathrm{r}} = n\pi a^2$ into Eq. (2.4) gives

$$N = \frac{WL}{2\pi a^3 p_{\mathrm{m}}} \tag{2.15}$$

Semispherical wear debris with radius a is generated in the probability k during contacts. The wear volume V in sliding distance L reads:

$$V = kN\frac{2\pi a^3}{3} = \frac{k}{3}\frac{WL}{p_{\mathrm{m}}} \tag{2.16}$$

The equation for the wear volume V indicates that the wear volume is to proportional to load and sliding distance, and is inversely proportional to hardness.

Abrasive wear is to remove softer material by asperity or debris with harder material during sliding. Cutting and polishing are established by the abrasive wear mechanism. In the case where softer surface is rubbed away by harder surface, the action is called 'two-body abrasive wear'. In the case where the surface is removed by harder particles such as debris particles and slurry, the action is called 'three-body abrasive wear'.

One of the simplest model for abrasive wear is shown in Fig. 2.5.

A rigid cone is penetrated into a surface with depth d. The cone is moved from left to right removing the surface. The load W is expressed as follows.

$$W = \pi\,(d\tan\theta)^2\,\frac{p_{\mathrm{m}}}{2} \tag{2.17}$$

where ϑ is the semi vertical angle of the cone. The wear volume V after moving the distance L reads:

$$V = d^2\tan\theta L = \frac{2\cot\theta}{\pi p_{\mathrm{m}}}WL = \frac{2\cot\theta}{\pi}\frac{WL}{p_{\mathrm{m}}} \tag{2.18}$$

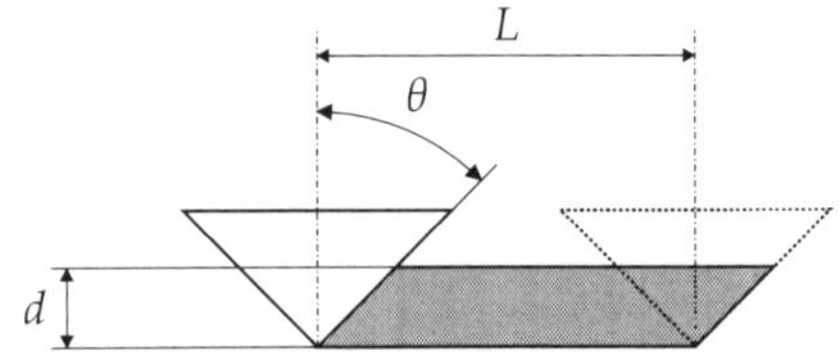

Figure 2.5 Model of abrasive wear.

According to Eq. (2.18), the wear volume by abrasive wear is the same trend as that in the case of adhesive wear. The volume is proportional to load and sliding distance, and is inversely proportional to hardness.

Corrosive wear [5] occurs as a result of chemical reaction of surfaces to surroundings such as lubricant, additives and atmosphere. If corrosion occurs to produce a film on its surface, the film is easy to be removed under sliding contacts. As a result, nascent surface is exposed to cause further corrosion. This process is repeated under activated circumstance, the wear volume is increased. Oxidative wear is one of types of corrosive wear and is cause by oxidative reaction. Oxygen is included in lubricant as well as atmosphere.

Corrosive wear possesses actions to create protected layer on its surface as well as to accelerates to produce wear volume. For example, in vacuum, friction is significantly higher compared to in air and depend on material of the surface because in air an oxidative layer could prevent from direct contacts of mating surfaces to weaken adhesive force. Extreme-pressure agent is used to create protected layers on the surface by corrosive action in engine oils. CMP process utilises effectively the combination of corrosive wear and abrasive wear.

Erosive wear is caused by the impact of particles such as solid and liquid to the surface. Erosive wear depends on impact speed angle, particles size and material of the surface and particle. Figure 2.6 shows the schematic result for the influence of the impact angle. The angle of 90 degrees means that particles are impacted in normal direction. At low impact angles, the wear volume is small for brittle materials while the volume is high for ductile materials. This is because abrasive wear occurs in the horizontal direction for ductile materials at low impact angles. At high impact angles, crack generation and propagation are the main part of wear for brittle materials. Therefore, at high impact angles the wear volume for brittle materials is higher than that for ductile materials. The size of particles also play an important role in mechanism of erosive wear. As the size of particles increases, the mode of erosion changes from ductile to brittle [6].

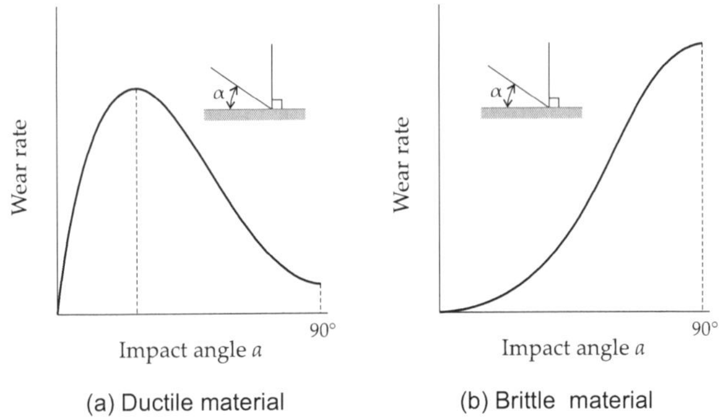

Figure 2.6 Schematic of variation in erosion rate for various impact angles.

Cavitation erosion is caused by the impact of liquid, which is the collapse of bubbles in lubricant. When bubbles collapse during shot period, significant high pressure from 100 MPa to 1 GPa is generated. There are two types of cavitation for lubricated areas. One is vapour cavitation. If the pressure is reduced down to the vapour pressure of liquid, the liquid evaporates to form bubbles. The other is gaseous cavitation. If the pressure is reduced, dissolved gas is released to form cavitation. For hydraulic systems, this type of cavitation is called 'aeration' [7]. In the water case, the vapour pressure is higher than the gas released pressure. Therefore, cavitation in water is vapour cavitation. In the lubricant case, bubbles are formed by the release of dissolved gas from the lubricant because the vapour pressure is lower than the gas released pressure. The shrink speed of bubbles formed by gaseous cavitation is not fast because released gas dissolves slowly into the lubricant. Therefore, cavitation erosion hardly occurs in the lubricant case while significant damage is found on the surface in the water case.

2.4 Lubrication

The function of lubrication is to separate mating surfaces with relative motion by a film to support load. In the case where the film is thick, a hydrodynamic force generated by the viscous flow

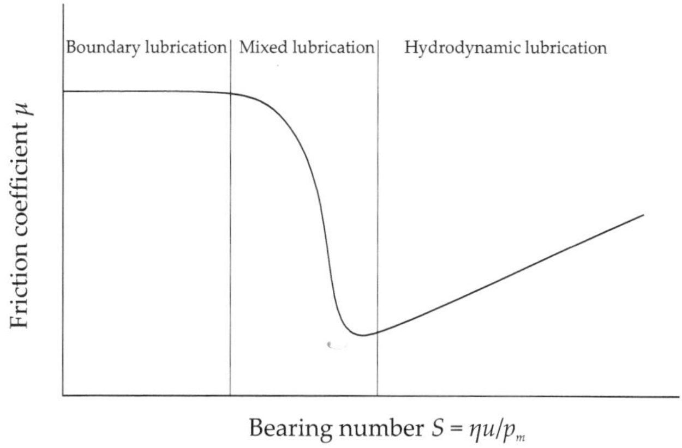

Figure 2.7 Stribeck curve.

separates the mating surfaces. This type of lubrication is called 'hydrodynamic lubrication'. Normally, liquid lubricant is used to achieve hydrodynamic lubrication. Gaseous could also produce hydrodynamic lubrication force because gaseous also have viscosity. The shear stress of lubricant is significantly low compared to that by solid–solid contacts. Wear is also expected to be so small because of prevention of solid–solid contacts. Therefore, safe and high efficiency operation with low friction and wear can be achieved in the hydrodynamic lubrication region. Figure 2.7 shows the Stribeck curve to indicate the lubrication region. The horizontal axis indicates the bearing number S defined as $S = \eta u/p_{\mathrm{m}}$, where η is the viscosity, u is the sliding speed and p_{m} is the nominal pressure. When the bearing number is high, that is, the nominal pressure is small, sliding speed is high and viscosity is high, the film thickness and friction coefficient are increased. If the film thickness decreases as a result of decreasing the bearing number, the friction coefficient starts to raise. This arises from starting direct contacts of the mating surfaces. The friction coefficient increases with further decreasing the bearing number.

This lubrication region is mixed lubrication. In the mixed lubrication region, the applied load is supported by the hydrodynamic force and direct contacts of the surfaces. When the bearing number is low, the friction coefficient becomes high and is independent to the bearing number. The lubrication region is called 'boundary lubrication'. In boundary lubrication, hydrodynamic lubrication force ceases, while direct contacts of the solid surfaces support the load. Additives in lubricant play an important role in characteristics of lubrication. Mono or a few layers of additives adsorbed on the surface decreases adhesive force to support the load [2].

The principle of hydrodynamic lubrication can be explained by hydrodynamic theory. The flow of lubricant is viscous flow in an almost parallel film, of which the thickness is significantly smaller than the length of the lubricated area. The flow can be expressed by the Reynolds equation [8], which is a simplified and combined one of the Navier–Stokes equations and continuity equation on the basis on some assumptions.

$$\frac{\partial}{\partial x}\left(\frac{\rho h^3}{12\eta}\frac{\partial p}{\partial x}\right)+\frac{\partial}{\partial z}\left(\frac{\rho h^3}{12\eta}\frac{\partial p}{\partial z}\right)=\frac{(u_1+u_2)}{2}\frac{\partial(\rho h)}{\partial x}+\frac{\partial(\rho h)}{\partial t} \quad (2.19)$$

where x and z are the coordinates of the sliding direction and its normal direction, t is time, ρ is the density of lubricant, p is the hydrodynamic pressure and u_1 and u_2 are the moving velocities of the surfaces. The two terms in the left hand side indicate the Poiseuille flow caused by the pressure difference between two distance. The first term in the right hand side indicates the Couette flow caused by the shear force. The second term describes the squeeze action between the surfaces. The principle of pressure generation in hydrodynamic lubrication can be explained as shown in Fig. 2.2. As lubricant is dragged from a wider space into a narrow space by the moving surface from left to right, pressure is generated to produce the Poiseuille flow so that the mass conservation of flow can be satisfied.

In a simple case of infinitely fixed pad bearings, the incompressible Reynolds equation can analytically be solved [9, 10]. Dimensionless forms of the Reynolds equation in steady-state conditions and film thickness read:

$$\frac{d}{dX}\left(H^3\frac{dP}{dX}\right)=\frac{dH}{dX} \quad (2.20)$$

$$H=1+K(1-X) \quad (2.21)$$

where K is the convergence ratio and X is the dimensionless coordinate defined as follows:

$$K = \frac{h_1 - h_0}{h_0} \tag{2.22}$$

$$X = \frac{x}{b} \tag{2.23}$$

where h_0 is the minimum film thickness and h_1 is the maximum film thickness. The dimensionless solutions of pressure P, load W and friction F are as follows:

$$P = \frac{h_0^2}{6u\eta b} p = \frac{1}{K}\left(-\frac{1}{H} + \frac{1}{H^2}\frac{(K+1)}{(K+2)} + \frac{1}{(K+2)}\right) \tag{2.24}$$

$$W = \frac{h_0^2}{6u\eta b^2} w = \frac{1}{K}\left(-\ln(K+1) + \frac{2K}{K+2}\right) \tag{2.25}$$

$$F = \frac{h_0}{u\eta b} f = \frac{6}{K+2} - \frac{4\ln(K+1)}{K} \tag{2.26}$$

These solutions are function of only the convergence ratio K. The maximum value of load is obtained at the convergence ratio K of 1.2.

References

1. Rabinowicz E (1995) *Friction and Wear of Materials*, 2nd ed, John Wiley & Sons, New York, NY.
2. Bowdon FP, Tabor D (1950) *The Friction and Lubrication of Solids*, Clarendon Press, Oxford.
3. Tabor D (1959) Junction growth in metallic friction: The role of combined stresses and surface contamination, *Proc R Soc Lond Ser A*, **251**(1266), 378–393.
4. Archard JF (1953). Contact and rubbing of flat surface, *J Appl Phis*, **24**(8), 981–988.
5. Rengstorff GW, Miyoshi K, Buckley DH (1986) Interaction of sulfuric acid corrosion and mechanical wear of iron, *ASLE Trans*, **29**, 43–51.
6. Sheldon GL, Finnie I (1966) On the ductile behaviour of normally brittle materials during erosive cutting, *Trans ASME*, **88B**, 387–392.
7. Hayward ATJ (1960) Aeration in hydraulic systems—Its assessment and control, Proccedings of Oil Hydraulic Conference, *Inst Mech Engrs*, 216–224.

8. Reynolds O (1886) On the theory of lubrication and its application to Mr. Beauchamp Tower's experiments, including an experimental determination of the viscosity of olive oil, *Phil Trans R Soc Lond*, **177**, 157–234.
9. Cameron A (1966) *The Principles of Lubrication*, Longmans Green & Co Ltd, London.
10. Stachowiak GW, Batchelor AW (2005) *Engineering Tribology*, 3rd ed, Elsevier Inc., Amsterdam.

Chapter 3

Articular Cartilage

Makoto Sakamoto
Department of Health Sciences, Niigata University School of Medicine, 2-746 Asahimachi, Niigata 951-8518, Japan
sakamoto@clg.niigata-u.ac.jp

3.1 Introduction

Articular cartilage is a connective tissue at the ends of the subchondral bone in diarthrodial joints. It does not have a blood supply, lymphatic drainage or a connection to nerves. The specific microstructure and composition of articular cartilage is thought to give the tissue its remarkable mechanical properties and durability. Articular cartilage provides almost frictionless joint motion and it absorbs and distributes the applied load to reduce localised stress concentrations in the underlying bone.

3.2 Structure of Articular Cartilage

The thickness of cartilage varies from 0.1 mm to 0.5 mm (rabbit knee joints) to 1.0 mm to 6.0 mm (human knee joints), and this variation

Hydrated Materials: Applications in Biomedicine and the Environment
Edited by Yoshitaka Nakanishi

ISBN 978-981-4463-22-5 (Hardcover), 978-981-4463-23-2 (eBook)
www.panstanford.com

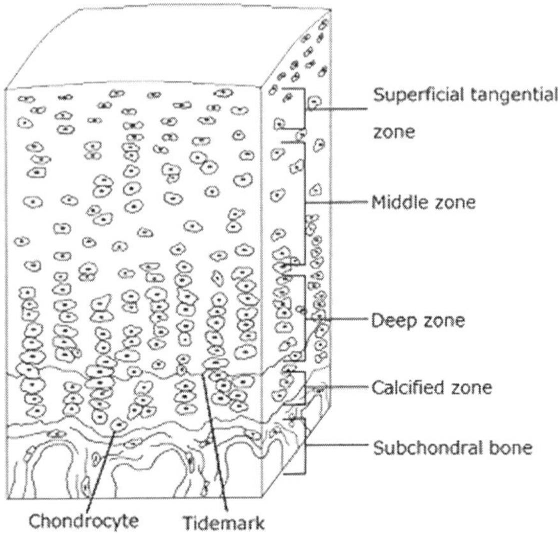

Figure 3.1 The structure of articular cartilage.

depends on the species, joints, location within the joints and age [1–4].

Articular cartilage is composed of a solid phase saturated with interstitial fluid (70–80% by wet weight) and mobile ions. The solid phase consists of cartilage cells (chondrocytes), sparsely distributed (1–10% by volume) within a fluid-filled extracellular matrix that is composed mainly of collagens and proteoglycans. The material properties of cartilage depend primarily on the properties of the extracellular matrix. The components of articular cartilage are not uniformly distributed in the matrix. Instead, cartilage can be divided into four zones: superficial, middle, deep and calcified, as shown in Fig. 3.1. The superficial articular zone is the thinnest one and forms the gliding surface of the joint. This zone is characterised by high water content (85%), relatively low quantities of proteoglycan, flattened chondrocytes and high quantities of collagen fibrils arranged parallel to the articular surface. The middle zone, in contrast, has round chondrocytes, the highest level of proteoglycan among the four zones and a random arrangement of collagen. The deep zone is characterised by collagen fibres with the largest diameters arranged perpendicular to the subchondral bone, columns of chondrocytes arrayed along the axis of fibril orientation and lower water content (approximately 60%). The calcified zone is partly mineralised and is the transition layer between cartilage and underlying bone. From a biomechanical perspective, the highly organised collagen network and the charged proteoglycans network are the most important components in the articular cartilage [3].

3.3 Mechanical Model of Articular Cartilage

The earliest model of the mechanical response of cartilage represented its matrix as perfectly elastic material [5]. To study the mechanical properties of cartilage and analyse the indentation of the tissue's matrix, Hayes et al. [6] and Sakamoto et al. [7] developed a linear elastic mathematical model in which the cartilage was modelled as an infinite elastic layer bonded to a rigid foundation and indented with rigid cylindrical and spherical indenters, as shown in Fig. 3.2. Based on viscoelastic theory, a simple model was proposed in which the cartilage layer was essentially a two-dimensionally distributed series of springs and dashpots and included a representation of the flow of fluid between the cartilage layers to account for inhomogeneity [8].

Mow et al. [9] proposed biphasic theory based on mixture theory to explain cartilage deformational behaviour where cartilage is considered to be made up of two immiscible phases: a fluid phase and a solid phase. The fluid phase representing the interstitial fluid is incompressible and inviscid, and the solid phase representing collagen fibres, proteoglycans and other components is porous, permeable and incompressible. The compressive deformational characteristics of the cartilage are due to the fluid flow and exudation through the porous, permeable solid. The rate of volumetric discharge Q across area A is related to permeability co-efficient k by Darcy's law [3]:

$$Q = kA\Delta P/h \tag{3.1}$$

where ΔP is the pressure gradient and h is the specimen thickness. The value of k ranges from 10–15 to 10–16 m^4/Ns and is inversely

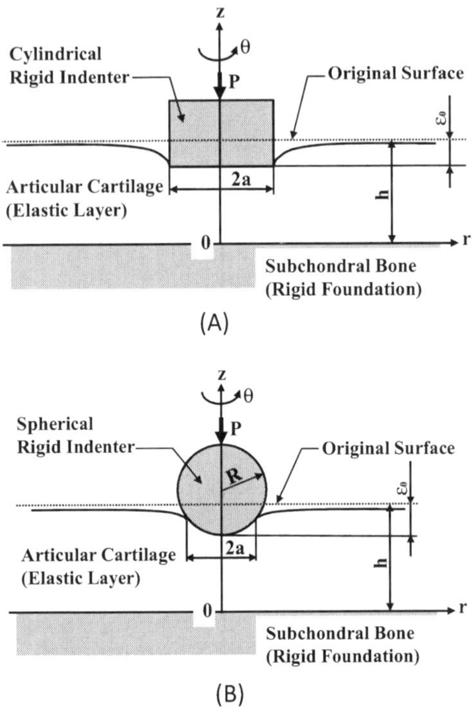

Figure 3.2 Indentation on layered materials with (A) a flat-ended cylindrical indenter; (B) a spherical indenter. The elastic layers are either bonded to the rigid foundation or freely laid over the foundation [7].

related to diffusive drag coefficient K by the following equation:

$$K = (\phi^f)^2/k \tag{3.2}$$

where ϕ^f is the tissue porosity, which is the ratio of the fluid volume to total tissue volume; its value is approximately 0.75. From this discussion [3], it is clear that the value of K will be very high and is in the range 10^{14} to 10^{15} Ns/m^4.

3.4 Lubrication Model of Articular Cartilage

Several theories describing the mechanisms of lubrication within synovial joints have been proposed [10]. Factors critical to the mechanisms of lubrication are the normal and tangential forces on the articulating tissues, the relative rate of tangential motion between these surfaces and the time history of both loading and motion [11]. A number of physicochemical modes of lubrication occur in synovial joints and have been classified as fluid pressure/film or boundary [10].

Several types of fluid-mediated lubrication modes exist. One type is hydrostatic. At the onset of loading and typically for a prolonged duration, the interstitial fluid within cartilage becomes pressurised; due to the biphasic nature of the tissue; fluid may also be forced into the asperities between articular surfaces through a weeping mechanism [12]. Pressurised interstitial fluid may therefore contribute significantly to the bearing of normal load with little resistance to shear force [3]. Moreover, at the onset of motion and/or loading, elastohydrodynamic and squeeze film types of fluid film lubrication can occur. In elastohydrodynamic lubrication, the pressure in the viscous film separating the surfaces causes significant elastic deformation of the sliding surfaces (compared to the surface roughness and film thickness). In squeeze film lubrication, the viscous lubricant is driven from between the surfaces being forced together in a normal direction. Additionally, in boosted lubrication, pressurised pools of trapped lubricant may contribute to the separation of cartilage surfaces as well [3].

In boundary lubrication, load is supported by surface-to-surface contact, and the associated frictional properties are determined by lubricant surface molecules. This mode has been proposed to be important because the opposing cartilage layers make contact over $\sim$10% of the total area, and this may be where most of the friction occurs [13]. Furthermore, with increasing loading time and dissipation of hydrostatic pressure, lubricant-coated surfaces bear an increasingly higher portion of the load relative to pressurised fluid, and consequently, this mode can become increasingly dominant [12]. Boundary lubrication, in essence, mitigates stick-slip, and is therefore manifest as decreased resistance both to steady motion and the start-up of motion. The latter situation is relevant to load bearing articulating surfaces after prolonged compressive loading [14] (e.g., sitting or standing in vivo). Typical wear patterns of cartilage surfaces [15] also suggest that boundary lubrication of articular cartilage is critical to the protection and maintenance of the articular surface structure.

3.5 Degeneration of Articular Cartilage

There is no known definitive cause of osteoarthritis (OA), and research suggests that there may not be one or a set combination of biomechanical and biochemical causes that leads to the progression of the disease. Damage to cartilage may be induced by the natural wear and tear of the matrix from decades of use, change in the general activity or lifestyle.

OA is characterised by an early onset of surface fibrillation, increased swelling, a decrease in stiffness, loss in tensile strength and an increase in tissue hydration and permeability, hypercellularity, followed by increased fissures, splitting and hypocellularity, penetration of blood vessels through the tidemark region, until the eventual wearing away to bone [16]. These characteristics have been linked to degradation in collagen, proteoglycans, chondrocytes [17] and lipids [18]. The swelling in OA is linearly correlated to the decrease in collagen [19]. With the decrease of the swell-limiting meshwork provided by the collagen fibrils, more water is able to bind to the proteoglycans, increasing tissue hydration and therefore the amount of swelling. The open spaces formed by the tangled collagen meshwork also provide for an increased permeability that is less frictionally resistant against the exudation of fluid. These factors lead to a decrease in matrix stiffness [19]. Mechanically, the cartilage would not be able to support the same static and dynamic forces as healthy tissue.

3.6 Conclusions

In conclusion, articular cartilage provides joints with low friction and wear resistance essential for repetitive gliding motion and shock absorption, while evenly spreading the applied load onto the underlying bone. The mechanical behaviour of this tissue depends on the interaction of its solid and fluid phases. Numerous factors can impair the function of cartilage and lead to OA. Mechanical factors are strongly implicated in the development of osteoarthritis, although the exact mechanisms are still not known.

References

1. Simon WH (1970) Scale effects in animal joints. I. Articular cartilage thickness and compressive stress, *Arthritis Rheum*, **13,** 244–255.
2. Ateshian GA, Soslowsky LJ, Mow VC (1991) Quantitation of articular surface topography and cartilage thickness in knee joints using stereophotogrammetry, *J Biomech*, **24**, 761–776.
3. Mow VC, Huiskes R (eds) (2005) *Basic Orthopaedic Biomechanics and Mechano-Biology*, 3rd ed, Lippincott Williams & Wilkins
4. Ateshian GA, Kwak SD, Soslowsky LJ, Mow VC (1994). A stereophotogrammetric method for determining in situ contact areas in diarthrodial joints, and a comparison with other methods. *J Biomech*, **27**, 111–124.
5. Elmore SM, Sokoloff L, Norris G, Carmeci P (1963) Nature of "imperfect" elasticity of articular cartilage, *J Appl Physiol*, **18**, 393–396.
6. Hayes WC, Keer LM, Herrmann G, Mockros LF (1972) A mathematical analysis for indentation tests of articular cartilage, *J Biomech*, **5**, 541–551.
7. Sakamoto M, Li G, Hara T, Chao EY (1996) A new method for theoretical analysis of static indentation test, *J Biomech*, **29**, 679–685.
8. McCutchen CW (1975) An approximate equation for weeping lubrication, solved with an electrical analogue, *Ann Rheum Dis*, **34**, 85–90.
9. Mow VC, Kuei SC, Lai WM, Armstrong CG (1980) Biphasic creep and stress relaxation of articular cartilage in compression: Theory and experiments, *J Biomech Eng*, **102**, 73–84.
10. Wright V, Dowson D (1976) Lubrication and cartilage, *J Anat*, **121**, 107–118.
11. Forster H, Fisher J (1999) The influence of continuous sliding and subsequent surface wear on the friction of articular cartilage, *Proc Inst Mech Eng H*, **213**, 329–345.
12. McCutchen CW (1966) Boundary lubrication by synovial fluid: Demonstration and possible osmotic explanation, *Fed Proc*, **25**, 1061–1068.

13. Morrell KC, Hodge WA, Krebs DE, Mann RW (2005) Corroboration of in vivo cartilage pressures with implications for synovial joint tribology and osteoarthritis causation, *Proc Natl Acad Sci USA*, **102**, 14819–14824.
14. Murakami T, Sawae Y, Ihara M (2003) Protective mechanism of articular cartilage to severe loading: Roles of lubricants, cartilage surface layer, extracellular matrix and chondrocyte, *JSME Int J Ser C*, **46**, 594–603.
15. Meachim G (1972) Light microscopy of Indian ink preparations of fibrillated cartilage, *Ann Rheum Dis*, **31**, 457–464.
16. Smith JO, Oreffo RO, Clarke NM, Roach HI (2003) Changes in the antiangiogenic properties of articular cartilage in osteoarthritis, *J Orthop Sci*, **8**, 849–857.
17. Goldring MB (2000) The role of the chondrocyte in osteoarthritis, *Arthritis Rheum*, **43,** 1916–1926.
18. Ballantine GC, Stachowiak GW (2002) The effects of lipid depletion on osteoarthritic wear, *Wear*, **253**, 385–393.
19. Bank RA, Krikken M, Beekman B, et al. (1997) A simplified measurement of degraded collagen in tissues: application in healthy, fibrillated and osteoarthritic cartilage, *Matrix Biol*, **16**, 233–243.

Chapter 4

The Human Skin and Hydration

M. Morales Hurtado, X. Zeng and E. van der Heide
Surface Technology and Tribology Group, University of Twente, Drienerlolaan 5, 7522 NB Enschede, The Netherlands
m.moraleshurtado@utwente.nl

4.1 Introduction

Human skin is the largest organ of the human body. It is an organic complex system that covers and protects the body from the external environment. Skin can be seen as a structured material composed of different layers. Each layer has a specific barrier function, such as to be a barrier against temperature changes, a barrier to ultraviolet radiations and microorganisms. Furthermore, the human skin has an important function in our immune system and it is crucial for our somatosensory system. A well-functioning skin is able to prevent excessive trans-epidermal water loss. There are hairline and exocrine glands, located in skin, which deliver hormones in order to adjust our body to environmental changes.

Skin also has an important sensory role associated with a group of sensory cells, an assortment of morphologically and functionally distinct mechanosensory cell types that are tuned to selectively

Hydrated Materials: Applications in Biomedicine and the Environment
Edited by Yoshitaka Nakanishi

ISBN 978-981-4463-22-5 (Hardcover), 978-981-4463-23-2 (eBook)
www.panstanford.com

respond to various mechanical stimuli, such as vibration, stretch and pressure. In glabrous skin of the palms and fingertips, Pacinian corpuscles, rapidly adapting Meissner's corpuscles, Merkel cell-neurite complexes, Ruffini corpuscles make up the majority of touch receptors [1, 2]. From the touch action, signals are produced by the sensory cells that are transmitted by the nerve system, through the spinal cord, to the thalamus and from there to the somatosensory part of the brain. Next, the sensory information is processed by the brain, that is, organised, identified and interpreted in order to fabricate a mental representation, which essentially determines the touch perception or tactility of a surface.

Furthermore, motor nerve fibres in the skin receive brain information in response to external stimuli and initiate responses such as exocrine glands secretion, relaxation or contraction of muscles and contraction or dilation of blood vessels.

The structure and behaviour of human skin is a well-researched area and is subject of many studies. Part of the research is directed to improving the comfort in areas, such as industrial engineering (furniture design, hospital clothes, sportswear and/or clothes in general), pharmacy and medicine (cosmetic research, wound dressings, drugs delivery systems, prosthetics, artificial skin and other artificial organs and tissues). The understanding of skin's mechanical, tribological and thermal performance is essential for the development of healthcare and lifestyle products that interact with the human body. This research topic has continuously attracted scientific studies over the past years and it is found that hydration has a large influence on the structure and behaviour of human skin.

4.2 Skin Structure

Human skin is a layered living tissue with a body area of approximately 1.8 m^2, an average volume of 3.5×10^{-3} m^3 and a weight with blood of 4.7 kg [3]. Each layer in skin show different properties as a function of its composition and its thickness range from a few micrometres in stratum corneum (SC) to the order of millimetre in epidermis and hypodermis.

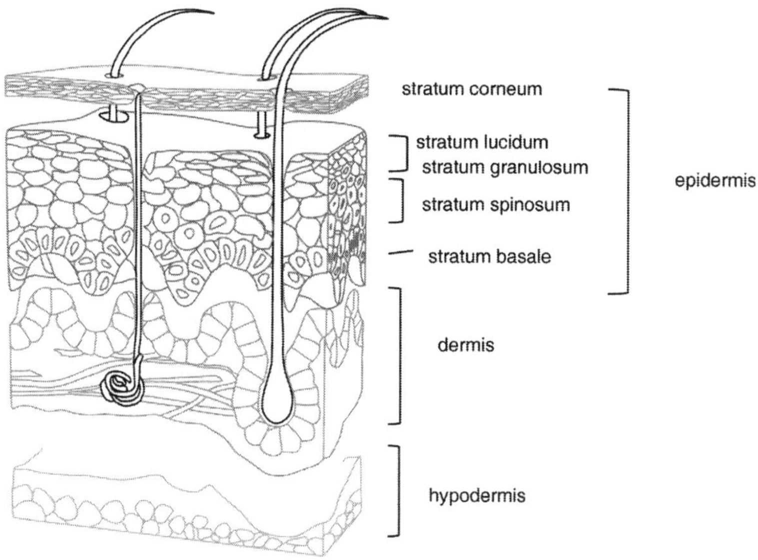

Figure 4.1 Main layers of the human skin structure and sublayers of the epidermis. (Illustration by Joe Lertola, image adapted and modified from *Skin Care and Cosmetic Ingredients Dictionary* by Varinia and DiNardo, Copyright © 2014.)

Properties of skin depend on the body site, age, hydration degree, use of creams and moisturizers, health and nutritional conditions that affect the skin conditions and hence, skin response after stress [4–17].

Basically, the structure of the human skin is composed of the following layers, as shown in Fig. 4.1.

4.2.1 *Epidermis*

Epidermis is composed of five different layers, SC, stratum granulosum (SG), stratum lucidum, stratum spinosum (SSp) and basal membrane (BM) and has a variable thickness between 30 and 130 μm depending on the body site.

SC is the outermost skin layer composed of dead cells from the differentiation process and has an important role in hydration control [18]. SC comprises a thin bi-phasic layer of about 10–20 μm frequently referred to as 'brick and mortar', where 'brick' regions consisting of corneocytes surrounded by the 'mortar' phase, which is an organised lamellar periodic bilayer of fatty acids, ceramides and cholesterol and water phases [19, 20].

The surface of SC is covered by an hydrophilic acidic film (pH 4–6) [3, 21] known as skin surface lipid film (SSLF) which results as a consequence of the mixing between sebum from the sebaceous glands secretion and lipids secreted by keranocytes. This film is composed of a complex mixture of triglycerides (42%), squalene (15%), wax esters (25%) and ceramides (25%) and shows a variable thickness depending on its locations on the skin surface [22, 23].

Cholesterol molecules located in the cellular membrane provides rigidity to the membrane and makes it less permeable to small polar molecules as water. Consequently, it helps to prevents water evaporation [24, 25].

Keratin is the major non-aqueous component of SC and seems to be the main factor responsible for the water storage and thus, in SC hydration [26].

Hence, the SC is a relatively impermeable film where some pathways provide water diffusion, oxygen diffusion and the passage of other compounds as moistures or creams. Specifically important in the mechanical behaviour of skin is water diffusion, which seems to occur primary by trans-cellular pathways where lipids presence are primarily responsible for the diffusive resistance [22, 27–30], see Fig. 4.2.

The progressive differentiation process of keranocytes from their origin in the basal stratum to non-viable corneocytes in the SC includes several intermediate steps in which the SG and the stratum spinosum are formed. The SG is critical for lipid synthesis [31], needed for crucial functions of the skin such as the control of water loss, the control of bacteria grow and the integrity with respect to physical–chemical protection.

4.2.2 *Dermis*

Dermis is composed of a tough, supportive cell matrix. It is a flexible connective tissue, containing ground substances, collagen and elastin fibres. The ground substance provides an environment of proteoglycans (PGs), glycosaminoglycans (GAGs), ions and an

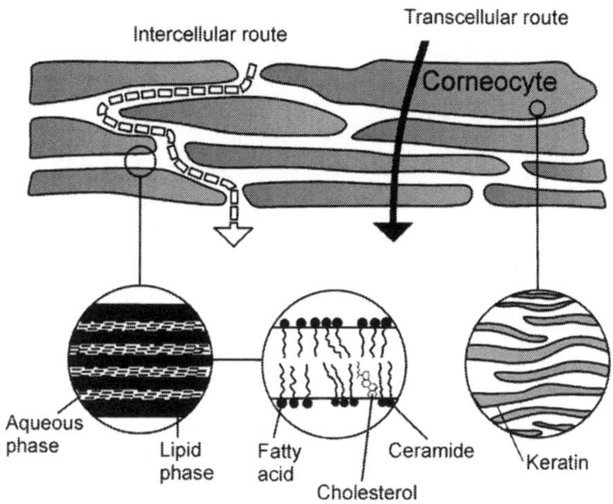

Figure 4.2 Intercellular and trans-cellular pathways for creams, moistures or other substances diffusion through stratum corneum. It shows water and lipid layout in the mortar phase, mortar composition and keratin distribution. (Image adapted and modified from *In Vitro Percutaneous Absorption: Principles, Fundamentals, and Applications* by Bronaugh and Maibach, Copyright © 1991.)

important amount of water, which imparts viscoelasticity and hydration to the skin. The specific composition of dermis provides strength and resilience to the skin. Dermis has a thickness in the range of 1–4 mm, varying with the body site. It is the place where blood and lymph vessels, nerves, sensory receptors, functional immune cells are located. Hair follicles, sweat and sebaceous glands also have their root in the dermis [5, 32].

4.2.3 *Hypodermis*

Hypodermis is the deepest layer of the human skin and is located between dermis and fasciae of the muscles. Small blood vessels, capillaries and fibroblasts form part of this layer, and adipocytes are embedded in a little amount of extracellular matrix (ECM) in this layer [5, 33]. The thickness depends on the body place. It protects muscles and internal organs against temperature changes and traumatic damage. The most important role of hypodermis is related to the storage of residual energy by lipid. Specific metabolic needs of the human body that, for instance, arise from sleeping and/or practicing sports are balanced by this reservoir of energy. The hypodermis has a role in hormonal functions as well [34].

It is reported that the role of the hypodermis in skin mechanical properties can be neglected [35].

4.3 Skin Properties

4.3.1 *The Hydration Characteristics of Skin*

The greatest amount of water in skin is located in ECM in dermis. Specifically, ground substance compounds are responsible for the water binding and hence, skin viscoelastic properties. Particularly, skin hydration is kept thanks to its chemical composition based on GAGs and PGs, respectively, which are able to establish links with water via hydrogen bonds and hence, are responsible for skin hydration degree and water binding. Later, water migrates to the upper skin layers and evaporates through the cellular pathways in SC while SSLF offers diffusive resistance to evaporation [36].

4.3.1.1 Dermis

Hyaluronic acid, heparan sulphate (HS), keratan sulphate (KS) or chondroitin sulphate among other complex molecules are some of GAGs and PGs present in the ground substance that are responsible for the vital hydration on the skin and hence, preserve skin's integrity [37].

Ground substance forms a tangled network of collagen, elastin, GAGs and PGs bound with water. As shown in Fig. 4.3, cells are located in this mesh. Since ground substance is composed of water absorbent molecules, its mechanical behaviour is a function of the water amount within it. Water is distributed in the ground substance in three different ways: an amount of water is taken up through the hydrogen bond with the hydrophilic groups of PGs and GAGs, knows as primary bound water. These water molecules are also next to the collagen and elastin chains. As water amount increases, mobility of collagen, elastin chains leads to the reorganisation of the structure. It

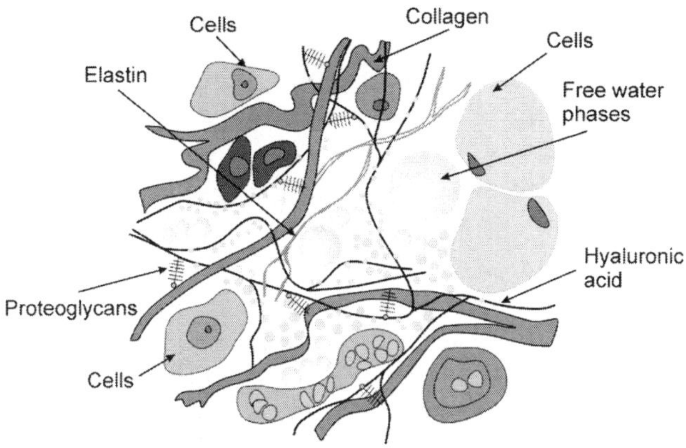

Figure 4.3 Water distribution into the ground substance. The image shows connective tissue compounds and water phases distribution: free water (big blue areas) embedded in the structure, drops of water next to the polymeric molecules (small blue circles) and other drops on the chains as linked water. (Image adapted and modified from Cummings, Pearson Education, Inc., Copyright © 2006.)

causes the secondary bound water process resulting in small water drops placed closest to the chains, but, not directly binding with them. Finally, the equilibrium state is reached, in which large water drops are formed in the polymeric network due to the coalescence of small water drops, see Fig. 4.3.

As a result, skin properties and its behaviour depend on the water uptake, which can not only modify the structure of skin, but also cause a decrease in its rigidity and modify its glass transition temperature. Water increase has a strong effect on the material and can modify at least in one order of magnitude the Young's modulus of skin [38, 39].

Aging has a strong effect on hydration of the skin. One of the problems related to aging is the decrease in GAGs and PGs located in the dermis. Furthermore, it is reported that the GAGs and PGS are subjected to structural changes with increasing age. Both aspects will alter the network properties of the ground substance [40], and consequently, change the distribution of water in the skin and change the hydration of the outermost layers. This could also be a reason for changes in skin mechanical properties with age [41].

4.3.1.2 Epidermis

Hydration of the human skin is not only possible due to the hydrophilic behaviour of GAGs and PGs that can retain water molecules within the ECM. The SC's composition and condition plays an important role as well [42]. SC not only acts as a relatively permeable barrier against water loss or chemical aggression, but also, SC has humectant capabilities important for maintaining its flexibility and control of desquamation. Keratin, corneocyte envelope (CE), lipids, desmosome and natural moisturizing factor (NMF) are the basic components of SC, which are important to maintain skin hydration. The chemical composition of saturated and unsaturated lipids from the mortar phase can be modified resulting in an alteration of the barrier properties and an increase of the trans-epidermal water loss through the skin [43, 44].

Consequently, micro-damaged SC and, specifically damage to its lipid content, reduces the SC's barrier function and promotes trans-epidermal water loss (Fig. 4.4). In line with this, Genina et al. [45] reported the reduced degree of hydration in damaged SC compared to undamaged SC.

4.3.2 *Mechanical Performance*

Research on the deformation behaviour of human skin, both with in vivo and in vitro skin, showed a specific mechanical behaviour of human skin as a function of the applied stress. This behaviour can

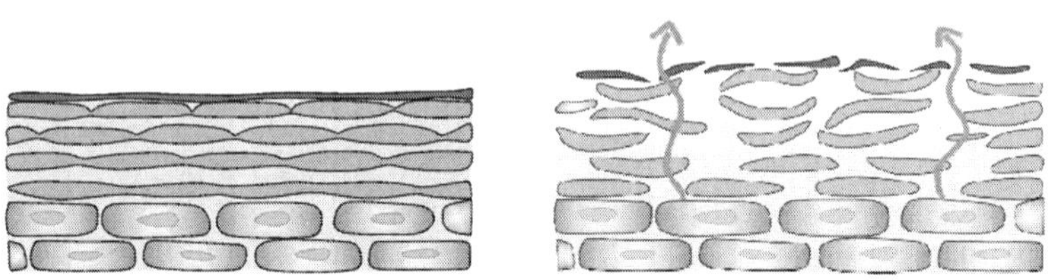

Figure 4.4 Structure of the stratum corneum in hydrated (normal) conditions (left) and in dehydrated conditions (right). The image on the right hand shows a loss of the cohesion between keranocytes and corneocytes, which causes trans-epidermal water diffusion outwards of the skin.

be summarised as anisotropic, non-homogeneous, non-linear and viscoelastic [46–48].

The mechanical properties of this complex structure can be represented by the ratio of the viscoelastic properties (U_v/U_e) and elastic ratio (U_r/U_f) to recover the initial position after stress. According to the nomenclature used by Agache et al. [48], the ratio of viscoelastic properties (U_v/U_e) is the delayed distension or viscoelastic creep (U_v) divided by the elastic distension (U_e), while the ratio of elastic properties (U_r/U_f) is the immediate retraction (U_r) divided by total deformation (U_f).

Basically, viscoelastic properties (U_v/U_e) depends on the ground substance [49], while elastic ratio (U_r/U_f) is correlated with the function of the elastic fibre network composed basically, of collagen and elastin. Figure 4.5 shows the typical curve for the deformation of viscoelastic materials.

$$\text{Viscoelastic ratio} = \frac{U_v}{U_e} = \frac{\text{delayed distension}}{\text{elastic distension}} \tag{4.1}$$

$$\text{Elastic ratio} = \frac{U_r}{U_f} = \frac{\text{immediate retraction}}{\text{total deformation}} \tag{4.2}$$

Theories of rubber elasticity (time independent) and viscoelasticity (time dependent) are typically used to explain and understand

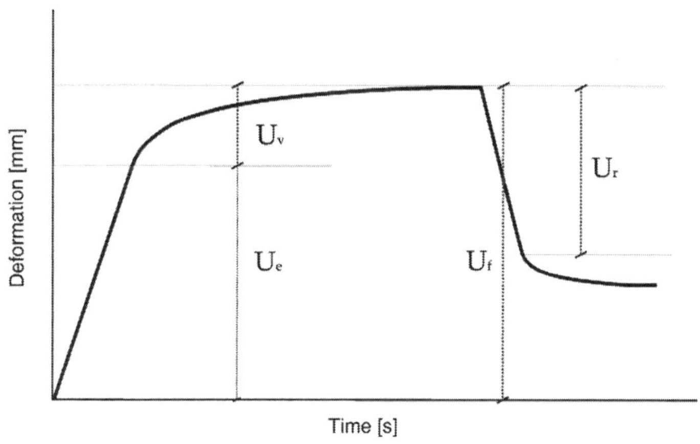

Figure 4.5 Deformation curve as a function of time for a viscoelastic material. Figure adapted from Ref. 62.

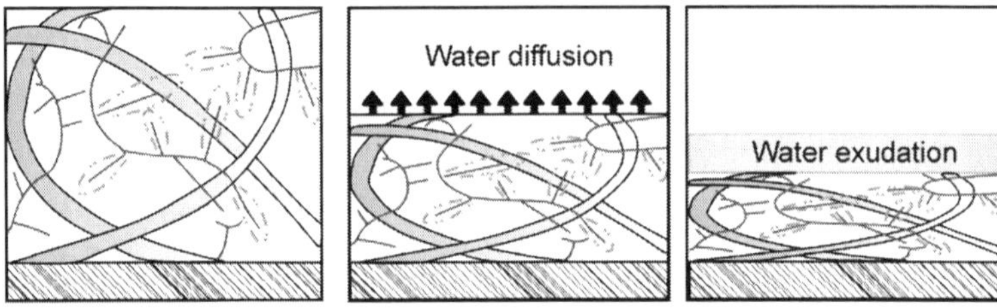

Figure 4.6 Interstitial fluid exudation after applied stress to the ground substance.

the viscoelastic behaviour of skin. The rubbery behaviour of skin can be explained from the collagen and elastin response while, viscoelastic properties characterised by creep behaviour and relaxation stress, appear due to the viscous resistance of the ECM components moving in the ground substance and water content diffusion, see Fig. 4.6.

Test methods with both in vitro and in vivo skin show a distinct difference in the mechanical behaviour of collagen and elastin. The first response to linear stretching of the skin is the deformation of the elastin. The contribution of the collagen fibres can be neglected in this first phase. In the second phase, collagen fibres start to stretch gradually as well, resulting in an increase of stiffness. Then, when all collagen fibres are stretched, the stress–strain relation becomes linear until high strain causes the fibres to rupture [50].

The specific composition of the ground substance gives rise to viscous behaviour. As a result, low molecular motions happen in the structure after applying stress, with a short characteristic time period. The complete rearrangements of water, fibres and other compounds occur at a longer characteristic time periods, resulting in viscoelastic material behaviour, which can be characterised by creep compliance and stress relaxation [51, 52]. The viscoelastic nature of the human skin, can be seen from the mechanical response, is as a function of time, temperature, hydration degree and the applied load. Although the composition of the dermis mainly controls the overall mechanical properties of the human skin, it is clear that surface related phenomena such as the tribological response are controlled by the epidermis, specifically the SC [53].

4.3.3 *Tribological Performance*

Surface properties of skin are important to solve dermatological problems, understand skin delivery mechanisms of cosmetics, improve ergonomics or establish a connection with the sense of touch. An important area of research related to the surface science of human skin aims at understanding the governing mechanisms for the skin friction. The coefficient of friction (COF) of human skin appears to be highly dependent on the hydration degree of skin, among other parameters that are related to the operational conditions and to the properties of the interacting surface. In fact, skin friction may be governed mainly by adhesion mechanisms [54, 55] when the hydration degree is minimal. This 'dry skin' condition results in skin behaviour independent of either velocity or load, as well as in a reduction of friction with increased surface roughness. Variations in hydration, sweat and sebum levels of skin can modify the frictional skin response. This introduces the need to consider the deformation related component of friction, that is, micro deformations caused by the interaction of asperities as well. The latter deformation component is a function of the hydration degree, sweat and the sebum film of skin [5, 8, 13–17, 38, 55–57].

Recently, Van Kuilenburg et al. [55] found a relationship between skin micro scale deformation and the frictional response underlining the need to consider micro deformations, both in dry and wet conditions, to be accurate in predicting frictional properties of skin. Masen [58] supports these results by showing an increase in the friction coefficient under hydrated conditions and intermediate roughness, which is in part attributed to the increased deformation of skin in wet conditions.

The SC hydration level seems to have an important relation with the elastic modulus at the micro scale, which is highly important from a tribo-mechanical point of view. Yuan and Verma [9] reported an elastic modulus of SC measured by nano-indentation between 100 MPa and 10 MPa in dry and wet conditions, respectively. The effect of humidity on the Young's modulus of SC was also examined by Park and Baddiel [10] who demonstrated that the mechanical properties of human skin depend on the water content. Specifically, they showed a Young's modulus decreased by 100 fold in the SC when the relative humidity (RH) increases from 60% to 100%.

Related to this, Peressadko et al. [11] mentioned the role of the spacing between ridges and asperities in elastic roughness surfaces, which can be applicable to the properties of skin. The importance of the shape and the surface texture (spacing parameters or waviness) in connections with skin tribology has also been reported by other authors [12, 13].

Despite the large number of parameters involved in skin frictional behaviour, it is clear that the frictional performance of human skin vary considerably among individuals. Actually, this is a consequence of the differences in skin hydration and lipid content of the skin surface as a function of the age and the anatomical region. For instance, aging causes significant changes in the hydration degree, arising changes in skin composition, mechanical properties and skin topography. Generally, these changes cause a decrease in skin elasticity ratio (U_r/U_f). The reduced hydration degree results in modified skin frictional properties, also associated to an increase in skin roughness and wrinkle formation [14, 15].

Hence as a result, aging skin becomes thinner, stiffer and less elastic with the passage of time and it undoubtedly has a role in the tribo-mechanical properties of skin [16, 17].

Additionally, differences in sebum content related to age have been found supporting the important role of the lipids content in the tribo-mechanical properties of skin due to its capability to avoid water loss and soften the skin [56].

Friction experiments with PTFE revealed that COF in sebum poor regions (and consequently considered hydrophobic regions) was considerably lower (COF = 0.19–0.25) than that measured on the sebum rich regions (hydrophilic, COF = 0.34) although the moisture content was comparable for both skin areas [17, 57]. Higher SSLF seems to cause changes in capillary phenomena resulting in increased adhesion while adhesion forces diminish if the lipid film is removed, as demonstrated by Pailler–Mattei et al. [57].

4.3.4 *Thermal Properties*

Skin compounds are affected by temperature changes. Since the human skin is a barrier between the environment and the interior of the human body, its interface controls the energy flux and

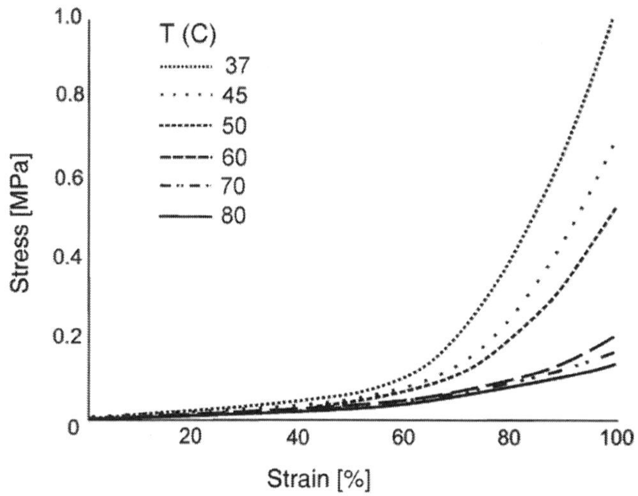

Figure 4.7 Stress–strain curve for skin samples at different temperatures (Figure adapted from Ref. 59).

contributes to maintaining a constant body temperature. Xu et al. [59] reported tensile and compressive properties of skin at different thermal conditions, showing the effect of temperature on skin. Their results show a decrease of the skin stiffness when the temperature increases, caused by dermal collagen denaturation, see Fig. 4.7.

4.4 The Effect of Hydration on Skin

4.4.1 *The Effect of Hydration on Skin Structure*

Water is crucial for maintaining the structure of the skin, thus ensuring its function and keeping its health and beauty. SC responds to external factors such as changes in humidity and facilitates biological protective strategies via signalling between epidermis and deeper skin layers [42]. Changes in hydration of the deepest layer of skin can be reflected in the changes of the properties of the SC as well.

Keratin, CE, lipids, NMF, desmosome and enzyme (Fig. 4.8) are important components of the SC. Changes to these components with

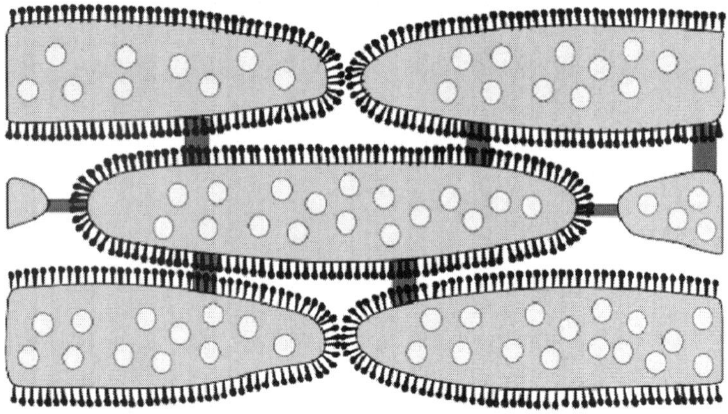

Figure 4.8 SC components. (Image adapted and modified from MD licensed to About.com Inc., Copyright © 2007.)

hydration are discussed and shown in Table 4.1 based on comparing dry and normal and/or hydrated skin.

The maintaining of an optimal level of hydration by the SC results in the formation of an effective moisture barrier by corneocyte strengthening, lipid processing and NMF generation. Firstly, lamellae lipid bilayer, organised predominantly in an orthorhombic packing state, provides an effective barrier to the passage of water through skin and reduces the rate of water flux. Secondly, the diffusion path length retards water loss because water must traverse the tortuous path created by the SC layers, corneocyte envelopes and desmosomes. Thirdly, NMF formed within the corneocytes retains water. In addition, enough water allows enzyme reactions that facilitate SC maturation events, together with corneodesmolysis and ultimately, desquamation [36, 60].

The influence of the hydration on the SC components further influences the corneocyte cell thickness and the appearance of the corneocytes. The corneocyte cell thickness increases linearly in a direction perpendicular to the skin surface with increasing hydration. Corneocytes are not swollen at low hydration levels (18–26% w/w), while at higher hydration levels (57–87% w/w), the corneocytes are more swollen in the central portion of the SC compared with the superficial and deeper layers [36].

Table 4.1 The effect of hydration on the SC components [36, 39, 42, 60, 61]

	Characteristics	
SC components	Dry skin	Normal and/or hydrated skin
Corneocyte envelope (CE)	Reduced CE maturation; fragile CE (CEf) predominates	Rigid CE (CEr) predominate in the more superficial layers, representing over 80% of the CE population; CEf are primarily in the deeper layers
Intercellular lipids	Total levels of ceramides decreased; levels of fatty acids increased. Reduction in phytosphingosine-ceramides; shortening and lengthening of acyl sphingoid based sphingosine and 6-hydroxysphingosine; increasing levels of oleate-ceramides. Lamellae bilayer: Chaotic, aberrant	High levels of ceramide 1 linoleate. Lamellae bilayer: Ordered; a balance between a solid crystalline state (orthorhombic packing) and gel (hexagonal packing)
NMF	Reduced NMF levels	NMF: 10% of the dry weight of the SC cells in well-hydrated skin
Desmosome	Intact desmosome, lipid disruption; Formation of visible, powdery flakes on skin surface	Total degradation of desmosomes and lipid structure; orderly and invisible process

4.4.2 *The Effect of Hydration on Skin Properties*

It is a trend that the skin frictional coefficient becomes higher when skin is hydrated compared with dry conditions [53, 54, 62–65]. Water is responsible for this increase due to the modification of adhesive forces that cause an increase in the contact area arising from the attraction of capillary bridges [57]. And, the increase in the friction coefficient is also attributed to the plasticising effect of water, leading to softened asperities on the skin surface and resulting in an increase in the real contact area (RCA) [55]. According to this, Derler et al. [66] reported low friction coefficients in dry (0.03–1.42) and higher in wet conditions (0.32–4.56) demonstrating the importance of hydration and surface topography properties of contacting materials.

Clearly, skin mechanical properties are strongly influenced by hydration and, hence, also depend on external phenomena such as temperature and relatively humidity and internal aspects related with body place and age [67, 68], see Fig. 4.8.

SC has a glass-transition temperature that shows changes in its mechanical and physical properties as a function of the temperature and as a function of the water content. As a result, the skin mechanical properties depend on humidity. At high hydration levels, the skin behaves more viscoelastic while, with low hydration or in dry conditions its elastic modulus is similar to a rubber [69]. As a consequence of changes in the properties of the SC, trans-epidermal water loss can be influenced negatively, causing changes in skin flexibility.

Papir et al. [70] confirmed the viscoelastic behaviour of the SC and the variability in its mechanical properties depending on the water content. They reported a great decrease in the Young's modulus of SC when the RH increases from 26% to 100%. Also, measurements on isolated human SC at several RHs showed that the elastic moduli diminished with the humidity increase from over 2 GPa at 30% RH to 3MPa at 100% RH [60]. Additionally, Levi [39] measured the elastic modulus of isolated SC after trypsin treatment placed inside a chamber with a controlled environment. Different RHs were applied by applying different saturated salt solutions and the ambient temperature and relatively humidity were monitored using a sensor. The results show and support previous data about the decrease in the mechanical properties of SC when it is hydrated, see Fig. 4.9.

These results give evidence for the predominantly elastic behaviour and for the high Young's modulus in dry conditions. Water content changes the mechanical behaviour of the SC samples to viscoelastic and the water content causes the Young's modulus to decrease considerably.

Correlation between SC–hydration and skin response has been also observed in tribological test samples with different roughness in hydrated and dry conditions. The results confirm the effect of the hydration on the length scale (reflected in surface properties as roughness) and show different skin response after hydration, which tends to increase the COF, albeit in a variable mode depending on the roughness. It stresses the important role of the forces that arise at the asperity level on the frictional response, for example, by

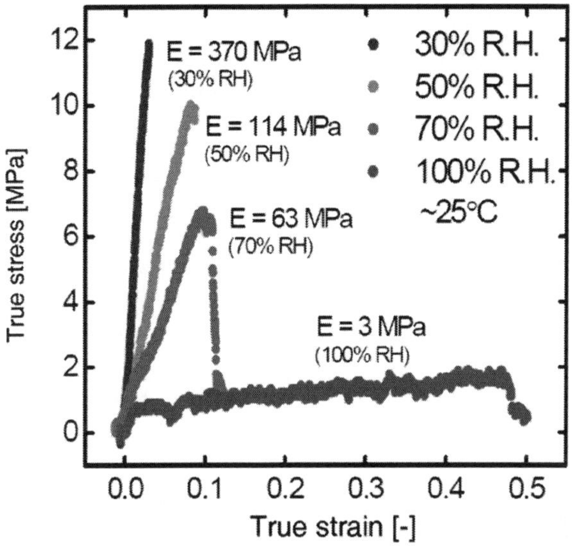

Figure 4.9 Stress–strain data of human SC showing the effect of the hydration on mechanical properties of SC [39].

increased deformation at the micro scale due to the softening effect of the hydration [58], see Fig. 4.10.

If both adhesion and deformation are considered important mechanism in order to determine frictional properties of skin then, the components of the friction force [58, 71, 72] can be seen as the sum of the forces required to break the adhesive bonds between the two surfaces at the asperity level, $F_{\mathrm{f,adh}}$, and the forces related to the deformation of the bodies in contact, $F_{\mathrm{f,def}}$. This concept was recently applied to the contact of a regularly patterned surface in contact with in vivo skin by van Kuilenburg et al. [73]. The regular pattern consisted of an array of summits of equal height with a common radius R_{summit} at a distance λ in both x- and y-direction, made by direct laser texturing. The term related to adhesion in the contact between the summits and the skin, is assumed to be proportional to the real area of contact for each summit individually, A_{real}, summit, see Eq. (4.3)

$$F_{\mathrm{f,adh}} = \tau A_{\mathrm{real,summit}} \tag{4.3}$$

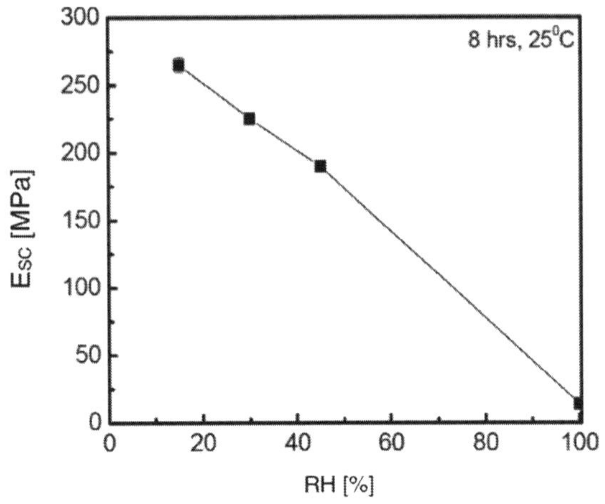

Figure 4.10 Elastic modulus of SC (E_{SC}) as a function of the RH [39].

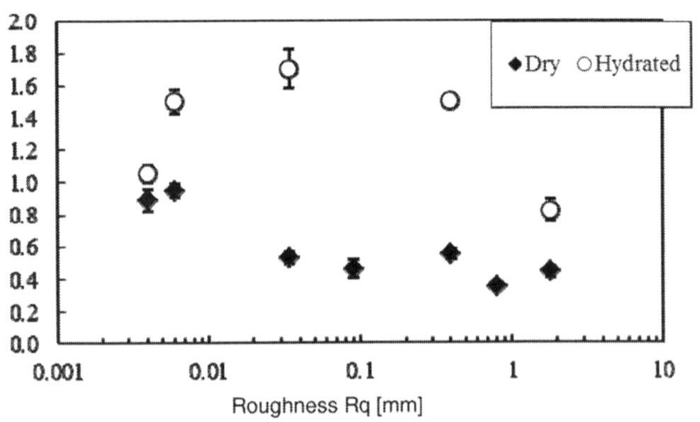

Figure 4.11 COF as a function of the surface roughness for hydrated and dry samples at normal load of 1 N [58].

The interfacial shear strength, τ, depends on subject specific or anatomical location specific 'lubricating' properties of the skin, like the sebum content, hydration of the skin, the amount of sweat, any effects due to treatments of the skin, such as the use of creams and conditioners [74] and possibly the hair density [75]. The deformation related term is assumed to be determined by the indentation of an individual summit into the skin, see Eq. (4.4) [76].

$$F_{\mathrm{f,def}} = \frac{3}{16}\beta\frac{a}{R}F_{\mathrm{n}} \tag{4.4}$$

in which β is the visco elastic loss fraction, a the radius of the contact area and R the radius of the individual summit present at the textured surface.

Expressions for the area of contact a_{H} and the indentation depth δ_{H} in the Hertzian case for an individual summit–skin contact are depicted in Eqs. (4.5) and (4.6), respectively.

$$a_{\mathrm{H}} = \left[\frac{3}{4}\frac{RF_{\mathrm{n}}}{E^*}\right]^{1/3} \tag{4.5}$$

$$\delta_{\mathrm{H}} = \left[\frac{9}{16}\frac{F_{\mathrm{n}}}{RE^{*2}}\right]^{1/3} \tag{4.6}$$

in which E^* equals the reduced elastic modulus given by Eq. (4.7):

$$\frac{1}{E^*} = \frac{1-\nu_{\mathrm{skin}}^2}{E_{\mathrm{skin}}} + \frac{1-\nu_{\mathrm{product}}^2}{E_{\mathrm{product}}} \tag{4.7}$$

with E_{skin} and E_{product} and ν_{skin} and ν_{product} the Young's moduli and Poisson's ratios of the skin and product surface, respectively at the asperity level.

Although the viscous character of skin is not incorporated in this contact model yet, it is possible to improve the quality of the model greatly by adding adhesion to the Hertzian contact model. As demonstrated by van Kuilenburg et al. [73], the normal force acting on an individual summit must be corrected to an effective normal force, $F_{\mathrm{eff,\,summit}}$ to correctly estimate the increased contact area for that specific summit–skin contact:

$$F_{\mathrm{eff,\,summit}} = F_{\mathrm{n}} + 2F_{\mathrm{adh}} + 2\sqrt{F_{\mathrm{adh}}(F_{\mathrm{n}} + F_{\mathrm{adh}})} \tag{4.8}$$

with the adhesive force F_{adh} based on the JKR theory of adhesion [77]

$$F_{\mathrm{adh}} = \frac{3}{2}\pi RW_{12} \tag{4.9}$$

The work of adhesion at the asperity level, W_{12}, gives the opportunity to fine tune the overall contact by tailoring individual summits to the presence of specific layers. The feasibility of this

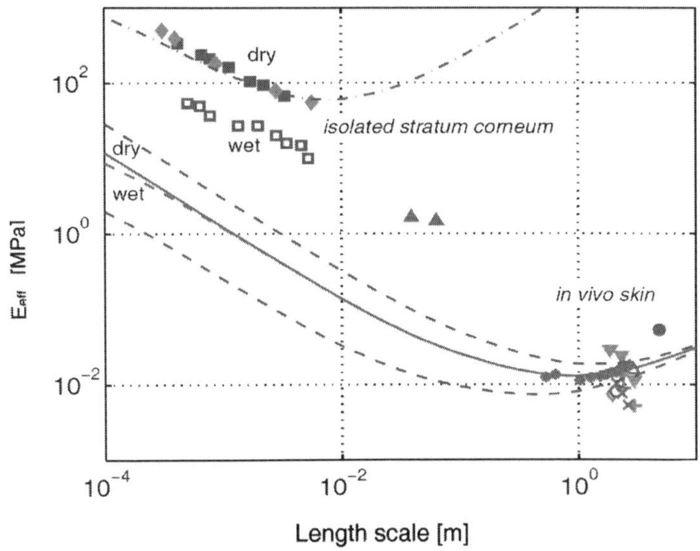

Figure 4.12 Effective Young's modulus (E_{eff}) for skin as a function of the length scale for dry and hydrated conditions [55].

approach however, is to be validated by future research. From Eqs. (4.4–4.9) one can construct an expression for the real or true area of contact, as a function of the material properties of the skin and product, as a function of the two controlling roughness parameters and the nominal contact area A_0, see Eq. (4.8):

$$A_{\text{real}} = \pi \left(\frac{3}{4E*}\right)^{\frac{2}{3}} \left(\frac{R}{\lambda}\right)^{\frac{2}{3}} \left(\frac{F_{\text{eff}}}{A_0}\right)^{\frac{2}{3}} A_0 \qquad (4.10)$$

By analysing the Eqs. (4.3), (4.10) and Eq. (4.5) it shows that there is an inverse relationship between Young's modulus and the total friction force, which implies an increased friction coefficient in hydrated conditions, due to the decrease in the Young's modulus.

Additionally, Van Kuilenburg et al. [55] recently showed collected Young's modulus data for human skin on various anatomical locations, from literature. Figure 4.11 shows the reported value of the Young's modulus on the y-axis and the length scale at which the value was measured on the x-axis. This indicates the influence of the Young's modulus in micro scale in both dry and hydrated conditions. These results also support the theory of the importance of surface

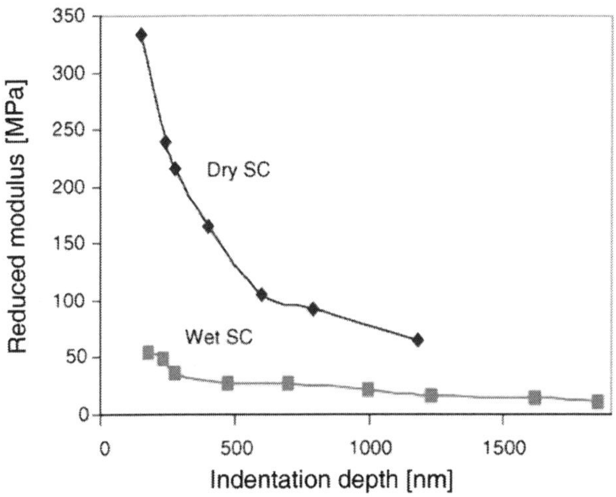

Figure 4.13 Reduced modulus for SC at different indentation depths [9].

roughness, shape and hydration on the tribo-mechanical properties of skin.

Yuan and Verma [9] also determined the elastic modulus (E) of isolated SC as a function of the depth using a nano-indenter. Elastic modulus as a function of the depth was calculated using the technique described by Oliver and Pharr [78], where the reduced modulus is defined as:

$$R_\mathrm{r} = \frac{\kappa_\mathrm{S}\sqrt{\pi}}{2\sqrt{A_\mathrm{c}}} \tag{4.11}$$

where k_s is the measured unloading stiffness *(dP/dh)* and A_c is the projected contact area.

The obtained results were plotted for dry and hydrated conditions and the curves (Fig. 4.12) shows the role of the hydration in SC of human skin while, in the inner layers the elastic modulus tend to be more similar with the increase of depth in both conditions. In this study, creep behaviour of the SC samples is also observed when the load was kept constant. This is a strong indication for visco-elastic behaviour.

Figure 4.13 shows the moduli obtained considering purely elastic deformations at 100 MPa for dry and 10 MPa for wet SC. The results are in line with the results of Papir et al. [70] who studied SC of

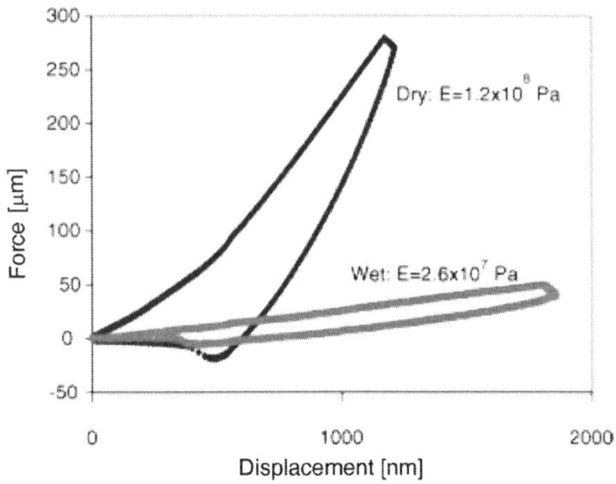

Figure 4.14 Force versus displacement for human SC in hydrated and dry conditions obtained by nano-indentation [9].

neonatal rats as a function of moisture content and at constant strain rate, observing a ductile transition at hydration levels higher than 70% RH.

To summarise, the presented results show a significant effect of hydration and of the length scale on the skin's mechanical behaviour and reveal the relative importance of the condition of the SC on the elastic modulus and corresponding frictional behaviour of skin.

4.5 Conclusions

The human skin is an organic complex system that covers and protects the body from the external environment. Skin can be seen as a structured material composed of layers with a specific thickness and composition. Hydration has a profound influence on the mechanical, thermal and tribological performance of the skin. Changes in hydration of the skin can be explained from changes in water content of the environment but, among other factors, also from changes to the concentration of PGs and GAGs in the dermis. The latter can be initiated by aging, causing, for instance, the appearance of wrinkles.

A large range of coefficients of friction and mechanical properties have been reported in the literature for the human skin due to its multi-layered viscoelastic structure, dependent on the degree of hydration. It is known that friction in healthy skin is strongly influenced by the state of the epidermis and SC which in turn depend strongly on the moisture content and the amount of sebum. The mechanical strength is determined mainly by the composition of the dermis: collagen, elastin and ground substance which is basically a network formed by water absorbent molecules bound with water.

From a tribological point of view, the adhesion part of the friction force is dominant in the friction response of dry skin. In wet conditions water has an important effect on the deformation of the skin layers at the micro scale. In wet conditions skin becomes softer and, hence, surface response can be due to both effects: deformation and adhesion.

Skin hydration is one of the essential parameters for understanding the mechanical, thermal and frictional response of human skin. Improved knowledge in this field will reduce the occurrence of specific dermatological problems and allows for the development of effective skin contacting products.

Acknowledgments

This work was partially supported by the Netherlands Ministry of Economic Affairs, the Provincie Overijssel and the Provincie Gelderland, by grant number PID 102050.

References

1. Johnson KO (2001) The roles and functions of cutaneous mechanoreceptors, *Curr Opin Neurobiol* **11**, 455–461.
2. Lumpkin EA, Marshall KL, Nelson AM (2010) The cell biology of touch, *J Cell Biol* **19**(2), 237–248.
3. Agache P, Agache PG, Humbert P, Maibach HI (2004). *Measuring the Skin—Non-Invasive Investigations, Physiology, Normal Constants*, 1st ed, Springer-Verlag, Berlin.

4. Hendriks FM (2005) Mechanical behaviour of human epidermal and dermal layers in vivo, Thesis, Technische Universiteit Eindhoven.
5. Silver FH, Kato YP, Ohno M, Wasserman AJ (1992) Analysis of mammalian connective tissue: Relationship between hierarchical structures and mechanical properties, *J Long Term Eff Med Implants*, **2** 165–198.
6. Lapière CM (1990) The ageing dermis: The main cause for the appearance of 'old' skin; *Br J Dermatol*, **122**(35), 5–11.
7. Tomlinson SE, Lewis R, Liu X, Texier C, Carré MJ (2011) Understanding the friction mechanisms between the human finger and flat contacting surfaces in moist conditions, *Tribol Lett*, **41**(1), 283–294.
8. Hendriks CP, Franklin SE (2010) Influence of surface roughness, material and climate conditions on the friction of human skin, *Tribol Lett*, **37**(2), 361–373.
9. Yuan Y, Verma R (2006) Measuring micro elastic properties of stratum corneum, *Colloids Surf B Biointerfaces*, **48**, 6–12.
10. Park AC, Baddiel CB (1972) Rheology of stratum corneum II. A physico-chemical investigation of factors influencing the water content of the corneum, *J Soc Cosmet* **23**, 13–21.
11. Peressadko AG, Hosoda N, Persson BNJ (2005) Influence of surface roughness on adhesion between elastic bodies, *Phys Rev Lett*, **95**, 124301.
12. Derler S, Huber R, Feuz HP, Hadad M (2009) Influence of surface microstructure on the sliding friction of plantar skin against hard substrates, *Wear*, **267**(5–8), 1281–1288.
13. Tomlinson SE, Lewis R, Carré MJ (2009) The effect of normal force and roughness on friction in human finger contact, *Wear*, **267**(5–8), 1311–1318.
14. Akazaki S, Nakagawa H, Kazama H, et al. (2002) Age-related changes in skin wrinkles assessed by a novel three-dimensional morphometric analysis *Br J Dermatol* **147**(4), 689–695.
15. Nakajima K, Narasaka H (1993) Evaluation of skin surface associated with morphology and coefficient of friction, *Int J Cosmet Sci*, **15**, 135–151.
16. Diridollou S, Vabre V, Berson M, et al. (2001) Skin ageing: Changes of physical properties of human skin in vivo, *Int J Cosmet Sci*, **23**(6), 353–362.
17. Cua AB, Wilhelm KP, Maibach HI (1990) Frictional properties of human skin: Relation to age, sex and anatomical region, stratum corneum

hydration and trans-epidermal water loss, *Br J Dermatol*, **123**(4), 473–479.

18. Tagami H, Yoshikuni K (1985) Interrelationship between water-barrier and reservoir functions of pathologic stratum corneum, *Arch Dermatol*, **121**(5), 642–645.
19. Bouwstra JA, Dubbelaar FE, Gooris GS, Ponec M (2000) The lipid organization in the skin barrier, *Acta Derm Venereol*, **208**, 23–30.
20. Lampe MA, Burlingame AL, Whitney J, et al. (1983) Human stratum corneum lipids: Characterization and regional variations, *J Lipid Res*, **24**(2), 120–130.
21. Eberlein-König B, Schäfer T, Huss-Marp J, et al. (2000) Skin surface pH, stratum corneum hydration, trans-epidermal water loss and skin roughness related to atopic eczema and skin dryness in a population of primary school children, *Acta Derm Venereol*, **80**(3), 188–191
22. Wertz P (1996) The nature of the epidermal barrier: Biochemical aspects, *Adv Drug Deliv Rev*, **18**, 283–294.
23. Elias PM, Cooper ER, Korc A, Brown BE (1991) Percutaneous transport in relation to stratum corneum structure and lipid composition, *J Investig Dermatol*, **96**, 495–499.
24. Finkelstein A, Cass A (1967) Effect of cholesterol on the water permeability of thin lipid membranes, *Nature*, **18**, 717–718.
25. Papahadjopoulos D, Cowden M, Kimelberg H (1973) Role of cholesterol in membranes effects on phospholipid protein interactions, permeability and enzymatic activity, *Acta Biochim Biophys*, **330**, 8–26.
26. Norlén L (2006) Stratum corneum keratin structure, function and formation – a comprehensive review, *Int J Cosmet Sci*, **28**, 397–425.
27. Elias PM, Cooper ER, Korc A, Brown BE (1991) Percutaneous transport in relation to stratum corneum structure and lipid composition, *J Investig Dermatol*, **96**, 495–499.
28. Potts RO, Francoeur ML (1991) The influence of stratum corneum morphology on water permeability, *J Investig Dermatol*, **96**, 495–499.
29. Suhonen M, Bouwstra JA, Urtti A (1999) Chemical enhancement of percutaneous absorption in relation to stratum corneum structural alterations, *J Control Release*, **59**, 149–161.
30. El Maghraby GM, Barry BW, Williams AC (2008) Liposomes and skin: From drug delivery to model membranes, *Eur J Pharm Sci*, **34**, 203–222.
31. Monger DJ, Williams ML, Feingold KR, Brown BE, Elias PM (1988). Localization of sites of lipid biosynthesis in mammalian epidermis, *J Lipid Res*, **29**, 603–612.

32. Edwards C, Marks R (1995) Evaluation of biomechanical properties of human skin, *Clin Dermatol*, **13**, 375–380.
33. Avram AS, Avram MM, James WD (2005) Subcutaneous fat in normal and diseased states: 2. Anatomy and physiology of white and brown adipose tissue, *J Am Acad Dermatol*, **53**(4), 671–683.
34. Ramsay TG (1996) Fat cells, *Endocrinol Metab Clin North Am*, **25**(4), 847–870.
35. Delalleau A (2008) Skin mechanical properties analyses through ultrasound imaging and inverse identification, *Proceedings of the XI International Congress and Exposition*, June 2–5, 2008 Orlando, FL.
36. Rawlings AV, Harding CR (2004) Moisturization and skin barrier function, *Dermatol Ther*, **17**, 43–48.
37. Brandt KD, Palmoski M (1976) Organization of ground substance proteoglycans in normal and osteoarthritic knee cartilage, *Arthritis Rheumat*, **19**(2), 209–215.
38. Derler S, Gerhardt LC (2012) Tribology of skin: Review and analysis of experimental results for the friction coefficient of human skin, *Tribol Lett*, **45**, 1–27.
39. Levi K (2009) Biomechanics of human stratum corneum: Dry skin conditions, tissue damage and alleviation Thesis, Department of Materials Science and Engineering, Stanford University.
40. Lapière CM (1990) The ageing dermis: The main cause for the appearance of 'old' skin, *Br J Dermatol*, **122**(35), 5–11.
41. Brown CT, Vural M, Johnson M, Trinkaus-Randall V (1994) Age-related changes of scleral hydration and sulfated glycosaminoglycans, *Mech Ageing Dev*, **77**, 97–107.
42. Rawlings AV, Matts PJ, Anderson CD, Roberts MS (2008) Skin biology, xerosis, barrier repair and measurement, *Drug Discov Today Dis Mech*, **5**(2), 27–36.
43. Potts R, Francoeur M (1990) Lipid biophysics of water loss through the skin, *Proc Nat Acad Sci USA*, **87**, 3871–3873.
44. Scheuplein RJ, Blank IH (1971) Permeability of the skin, *Physiol Rev*, **51**(4), 702–747.
45. Genina EA, Bashkatov AN, Korobko AA, et al. (2008) Optical clearing of human skin: Comparative study of permeability and dehydration of intact and photo thermally perforated skin, *J Biomed Opt*, **13**(2), v 021102.
46. Wan Abas WA, Barbenel JC (1982) Uniaxial tension test of human skin in vivo, *J Biomed Eng*, **4**(1), 65–71.

47. Alexander H, Cook TH (1977) Accounting for the natural tension in the mechanical testing of human skin, *J Investig Dermatol*, **69**, 310–314.
48. Agache PG, Monneur C, Leveque JL, De Rigal J (1980) Mechanical properties and Young's modulus of human skin in vivo, *J Arch Dermatol Res*, **269**, 221–232.
49. Dulgerova P (2004) Biophysical modeling of viscoelastic deformations of cattle skin in vivo, *Trakia J Sci*, **2**(4), 1–3.
50. Daly CH (1982) Biomechanical properties of dermis, *J Invest Dermatol*, **79**(1), 17s–20s.
51. Dunn MG, Silver FH (1983) Viscoelastic behaviour of human connective tissues: Relative contribution of viscous and elastic components, *Connect Tissue Res*, **12**(1), 59–70.
52. Findley WN, Lai JS, Onaran K (1976) *Creep and Relaxation of Nonlinear Viscoelastic Materials*, 2nd Ed Dover Publication, New York, NY.
53. Lévêque JL, Audoly B (2013) Influence of stratum corneum on the entire skin mechanical properties, as predicted by a computational skin model, *Skin Res Technol*, **19**(1), 42–46.
54. Adams MJ, Briscoe BJ, Johnson SA (2007) Friction and lubrication of human skin, *Tribol Lett*, **26**(3).
55. Van Kuilenburg J, Masen MA, Van der Heide E (2012) Contact modeling of human skin: What value to use for the modulus of elasticity? *J Eng Tribol*, (0), 1–13.
56. Cua AB, Wilhelm KP, Maibach HI (1995) Skin surface lipid and skin friction: Relation to age, sex and anatomical region, *Skin Pharmacol*, **8**(5), 246–251.
57. Pailler-Mattei C, Nicoli S, Pirot F, Vargiolu R, Zahouani H (2009) A new approach to describe the skin surface physical properties in vivo, *Colloids Surf B Biointerfaces*, **68**(2), 200–206.
58. Masen MA (2011) A system based experimental approach to tactile friction, *J Mech Behav Biomed Mater*, **4**(8), 1620–1626.
59. Xu F, Seffen KA, Lu TJ (2008) Temperature-dependent mechanical behaviors of skin tissue, *IAENG Int J Comput Sci*, **35**(1), 92–101.
60. Rawlings AV, Matts PJ (2005) Stratum corneum moisturization at the molecular level: An update in relation to the dry skin cycle, *J Investig Dermatol*, **124**, 1099–1110.
61. Harding CR, Watkinson A, Rawlings AV, Scott IR (2000) Dry skin, moisturization and corneodesmolysis, *Int J Cosmet Sci*, **22**(1), 21–52.

62. Lévêque JL, Audoly B (2013) Influence of stratum corneum on the entire skin mechanical properties, as predicted by a computational skin model, *Skin Res Technol*, **19**(1), 42–46.
63. Gerhardt LC, Strässle V, Lenz A, Spencer ND, Derler S (2008) Influence of epidermal hydration on the friction of human skin against textiles, *J R Soc Interface*, **5**, 1317–1328.
64. Elsner P, Wilhelm D, Maibach HI (1990) Frictional properties of human forearm and vulvar skin: Influence of age and correlation with trans-epidermal water loss and capacitance, *Dermatologica*, **181**(2), 88–91.
65. Persson BNJ, Kovalev A, Gorb SN (2012) Contact mechanics and friction on dry and wet human skin, *Tribol Lett*, (accepted Nov. 2012).
66. Derler S, Gerhardt LC, Lenz A, Bertaux E, Hadad M (2009) Friction of human skin against smooth and rough glass as a function of the contact pressure, *Tribol Int*, **42**(11–12), 1565–1574.
67. Gitis N, Sivamani R (2004) Tribometrology of skin, *Tribol Trans*, **47**, 1–9.
68. Wildnauer RH, Bothwell JW, Douglass AB (1971) Stratum corneum biomechanical properties. I. Influence of relative humidity on normal and extracted human stratum corneum, *J Invest Dermatol*, **56**(1), 72–78.
69. Edwards C, Marks R (1995) Evaluation of biomechanical properties of human skin, *Clin Dermatol*, **13**, 375–380.
70. Papir YS, Hsu KH, Wildnauer RH (1975) The mechanical properties of stratum corneum I The effect of water and ambient temperature on the tensile properties of newborn rat stratum corneum, *Biochim Biophys Acta*, **399**, 170–180.
71. Boyer G, Laquièze L, Le Bot A, Laquièze S, Zahouani H (2009) Dynamic indentation on human skin in vivo: Ageing effects, *Skin Res Technol*, **15**, 55–67.
72. Wolfram LJ (1983) Friction of skin, *J Soc Cosmet Chem*, **34**, 465–476.
73. Van Kuilenburg J, Masen MA, Van Der Heide E (2013) The role of the skin microrelief in the contact behaviour of human skin: Contact between the human finger and regular surface textures, *Tribol Int*, dx.doi.org/10.1016/j.triboint.2012.11.024.
74. Ramalho A, Silva CL, Pais AACC, Sousa JJS (2007) In vivo friction study of human skin: Influence of moisturizers on different anatomical sites, *Wear*, **263**, 1044–1049.
75. Veijgen NK (2013) Skin friction—A novel approach to measuring in vivo human skin, PhD Thesis University of Twente, Enschede, The Netherlands.

76. Greenwood JA, Tabor D (1958) The friction of hard sliders on lubricated rubber: The importance of deformation losses, *Proc Phys Soc*, **71**, 989–1001.
77. Johnson KL, Kendall K Roberts AD (1971) Surface energy and the contact of elastic solids, *Proc R Soc Lond A*, **324**, 301–313.
78. Oliver WC, Pharr GM (1992) An improved technique for determining hardness and elastic modulus using load and displacement sensing indentation experiments, *J Mater Res*, **7**(6).

Chapter 5

Hydrogel Materials for Tissue Engineering

Berkay Ozcelik, Greg Guanghua Qiao and Geoffrey Wayne Stevens

Particulate Fluids Processing Centre, Department of Chemical and Biomolecular Engineering, University of Melbourne, Australia

gstevens@unimelb.edu.au

5.1 Tissue Engineering

Ever since Langer and Vacanti introduced the concept of tissue engineering [1], it has been a research field of high interest due to the possibilities it offers in addressing tissue and organ failure. Current treatments include administration of therapeutics, reconstructive surgery, organ transplantation and implantation of mechanical devices [1, 2]. However, these treatments have major drawbacks such as adverse side effects, donor shortages, transplant rejection and failure, mechanical failure as well as risks of major immune responses [1, 2]. In comparison, tissue engineering aims to address these issues via autologous regeneration or repair, to restore, maintain or improve tissue function [1]. A major component of tissue engineering research is the study and development of

Hydrated Materials: Applications in Biomedicine and the Environment
Edited by Yoshitaka Nakanishi

ISBN 978-981-4463-22-5 (Hardcover), 978-981-4463-23-2 (eBook)
www.panstanford.com

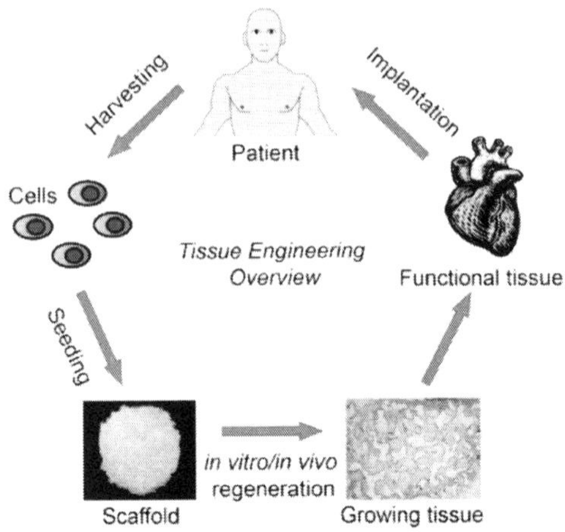

Figure 5.1 Tissue engineering overview.

scaffolds. Scaffolds are constructs that permit tissue regeneration while providing a suitable environment and mechanical support [3, 4]. The fundamental aim of tissue engineering involves seeding patients' cells that are harvested onto a suitable scaffold, whereby the tissue ideally regenerates into a functional tissue in vitro or in vivo (Fig. 5.1) which will then repair or restore the compromised function.

In this chapter we shall explore the types of hydrogels that have been used and their successes in a range of applications for tissue engineering. In choosing hydrogels for tissue engineering, both the biological and physical responses towards scaffolds and their physical properties need to be considered. These biological responses and physical properties can be vital in determining the success or the failure of a scaffold implant. Both of these are discussed in the following sections.

5.2 Cell and Tissue Responses

5.2.1 *Cell–Surface Interactions*

Most cells in the body are anchorage dependant and interact with their surroundings via 'bio-recognition' [5, 6]. This is achieved through the interaction between the receptors expressed on cell surfaces and the ligands such as proteins that are present on the material surface (Fig. 5.2) [5, 6]. When a material is implanted, proteins that are present in the surrounding area adsorb onto the material surface via hydrophobic and electrostatic interactions [6]. Depending on the surface properties of the material, proteins may denature once adsorbed. Denatured proteins are not easily recognised and can decrease the interaction between material and cells. Elbert and Hubble explain that hydrophobic surfaces allow for increased protein adsorption and can lead to the denaturation of the adsorbed proteins [6].

The interactions between the scaffold and tissues take place on the material surface [7]. As a result of this, scaffolds surfaces need to permit appropriate interactions with proteins in the surrounding environment and subsequently with cells. For example, the extent of hydrophilicity and hydrophobicity plays a very significant role. As described by Ma et al., if the hydrophobicity of a surface is too high then proteins that adsorb may denature, making it difficult for cells to interact with the surface [7]. A balance between hydrophobicity and hydrophilicity needs to be established for the best outcomes in terms of cell–surface interactions [7]. Denaturation of the proteins leads to the loss of their bioactivity, and since the interactions between cells and the proteins deposited on material surfaces are highly significant, such denaturation is undesirable (Fig. 5.2).

5.2.2 *Foreign Body Responses*

A major problem faced when implanting any material in vivo including scaffolds, is the foreign body response (FBR). As a result of the injury caused by the implantation procedure, increased blood flow leads to escape of proteins from the vasculature. Increase in protein concentration near the implantation site leads to further adsorption of proteins onto the material surface [8–10].

Following protein adsorption and the possible denaturation of these proteins on the material surface, macrophages attempt to phagocytose the implanted material. If the material is very large, macrophages fuse to form multinucleated cells known as foreign body giant cells (FBGC) (Fig. 5.3) [11]. FBGCs subsequently attempt

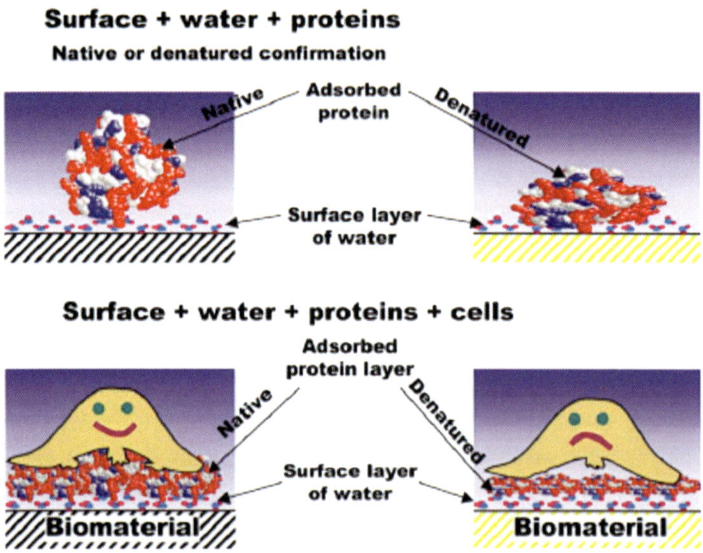

Figure 5.2 Cell–surface interactions with native and denatured proteins on material surfaces. Adapted from Ref. [5].

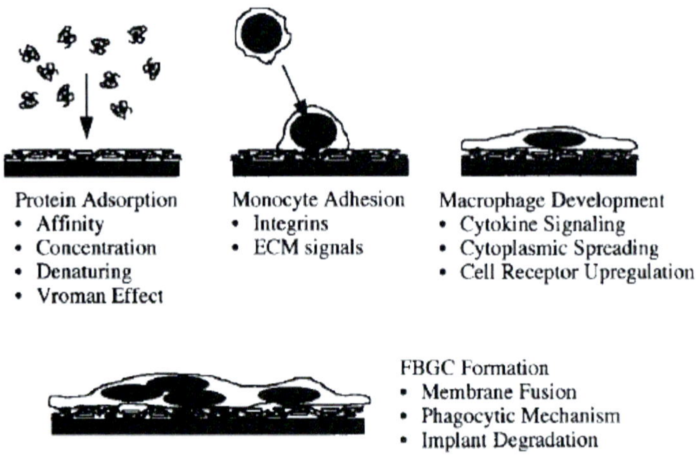

Figure 5.3 FBR and FBGC formation. Adapted from Ref. [8].

to degrade the material. If the material doesn't degrade rapidly, then fibrous encapsulation ensues [8–10], which prevents material interaction and integration by acting as a 'physico-chemical' barrier [10].

Brodbeck et al. and Anderson et al. conclude that hydrophobic and positively charged surfaces promote inflammatory responses and hydrophilic and negatively charged surfaces have anti-inflammatory properties [8, 9]. It has been described by Ma et al. that protein denaturation related to surface hydrophobicity is one of the major causes of FBR initiation [7].

5.2.3 *Vascularisation*

The penetration of cells and formation of vascular networks in a three-dimensional (3D) scaffold is crucial. These vessels allow the transport and delivery of nutrients and factors for the proliferation of cells and their survival [12].

Without the formation of an extensive vascular network, size of the tissue engineered constructs that can be obtained is significantly limited [13]. Vascularisation of a newly developing tissue or biomaterials in vivo takes place via angiogenesis or vasculogenesis [13].

Vascularisation of a developing tissue is essential for its survival and for the effective vascularisation of a scaffold construct, appropriate interconnected pore structures need to be present.

5.3 Tissue Engineering Scaffold Materials

With these biological responses in consideration, various types of materials have been studied for the fabrication of scaffolds. These materials are generally classified as being of synthetic or natural origin [14]. Natural and synthetic polymers possess advantages and disadvantages that determine their suitability for various tissue engineering applications.

5.3.1 *Natural Polymers*

Scaffolds derived from natural polymers can behave similar to the extracellular matrix (ECM) and possess desirable properties such as biocompatibility, biodegradability and inherent cell-scaffold interactions [14, 15]. Natural materials, including collagen, alginate, chitosan and hydroxyapatite, have been utilised to prepare scaffolds for tissue engineering applications [16–19]. Regardless of the many advantages, there are certain issues in regards to the use of naturally materials, such as variation in quality due to sourcing, risk of disease transmission and immunogenicity [20–24]. In addition, the processing methods required to obtain these natural materials can significantly affect their mechanical properties. For example, even though collagen demonstrates high mechanical strength in vivo, the process of harvesting, isolation and purification negatively impacts its mechanical properties through the loss of natural cross-links [25].

5.3.2 *Synthetic Polymers*

Employment of synthetic polymers to prepare scaffolds offers certain advantages over natural polymers, including good batch-to-batch consistency and a high degree of control and tailorability during the fabrication process [26]. Nonetheless, there are certain drawbacks, such as the use of organic solvents during synthesis [27]. Moreover, challenges in regards to cellular interactions arise since synthetic polymers lack the biological functionalities that are present in the ECM [14, 28].

Synthetic polymers including polyfumarates, polyurethanes, polyanhydrides and poly(α-hydroxy acids) have been explored as scaffold materials for a variety of tissue engineering applications [29–33]. Poly(α-hydroxy acids) such as poly(ϵ-caprolactone), poly(lactic acid), poly(glycolic acid) and their co-polymers are some of the most extensively studied polymers for scaffold fabrication [14, 34]. Poly(α-hydroxy acids) provide desirable physical and biocompatibility characteristics [35], however such polymers are very hydrophobic [36], which is a significant factor in FBRs [8, 9].

5.4 Hydrogels

5.4.1 *Hydrogel Tissue Engineering Scaffolds*

As a result of concerns regarding the use of hydrophobic materials, recent scaffold research is shifting towards the development of high water absorbing hydrogels [36]. A hydrogel can be defined as an insoluble 3D network that is held together by chemical or physical bonds [37]. The suitability of hydrogels for tissue engineering applications comes from their high water absorption ($\geq$10–20 wt% water) and similar physico-chemical characteristics to that of many tissues and the ECM [36, 37]. In addition, the mechanical strength and degradation properties of hydrogels can be altered by modifying factors such as the type and molecular weight of polymers used, cross-linking densities, porosity and fabrication conditions [36–40]. This allows hydrogels to be used as scaffolds for hard tissues, such as bone and cartilage, and soft tissues, such as fat and muscle. These hydrophilic networks have found a variety of potential applications in tissue engineering; either as scaffolds, cell delivery vehicles or tissue replacements.

Hydrogels can be synthesised from a variety of hydrophilic natural polymers; that is, collagen, chitosan and hyaluronic acid, and synthetic polymers; that is, poly(vinyl alcohol), poly(2-hydroxyethyl methacrylate) (PHEMA) and poly(ethylene glycol) (PEG) [41–54]. Synthetic hydrophilic polymers such as PEG (Fig. 5.4), have been explored for biomedical applications due to their low toxicity, minimal immunogenicity and anti-protein fouling properties [55–58]. The hydrophilic nature of hydrogels and anti-protein fouling properties are beneficial when trying to minimise FBR [7, 59]. This non-immunogenic property makes them advantageous as hydrogel scaffolds. Due to their anti-protein fouling properties, coatings

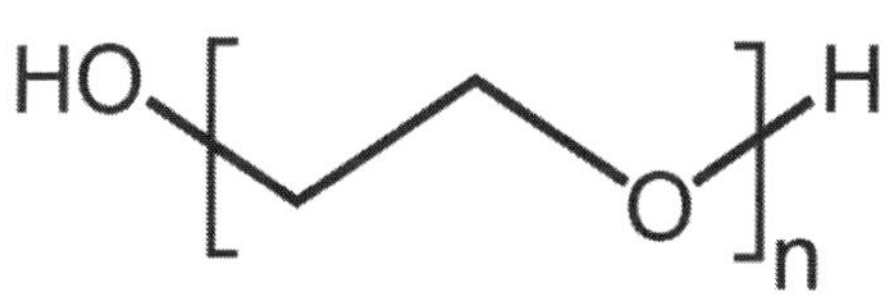

Figure 5.4 PEG chemical structure.

from materials such as PEG also prevent non-specific protein and bacterial binding on implantable material surfaces [60].

For example, as a US Food and Drug Administration approved polymer for certain applications [55], PEG has also been widely investigated as a material for tissue engineering applications [61]. In vitro and in vivo studies have demonstrated these desirable properties, as well as the cellular tissue penetration and vascularisation capabilities of scaffolds fabricated using PEG [62–65].

5.4.2 *Desired Hydrogel Scaffold Properties*

For ideal cellular interactions and tissue regeneration, scaffolds need to possess certain physico-chemical properties [3, 4, 14, 34] including (i) 3D structural support; (ii) an interconnected porous structure for cell and tissue penetration; (iii) suitable and controllable biodegradation rates; (iv) appropriate surface properties for cell–surface interactions; (v) low toxicity and immunogenicity of both the scaffold and its degradation products and (vi) good structural integrity for maintenance of the 3D shape during degradation and tissue regeneration [3, 4, 14, 34].

The desired physical and chemical properties of hydrogels are site specific and depend on the local tissue environment. A 3D, interconnected porous structure is required for the penetration and proliferation of tissue. The porous structure of a scaffold plays an important role in the integration of the scaffold with the surrounding tissue in vivo. Pore size and interconnectivity are significant factors in the migration, survival and proliferation of cells as well as nutrient transport and vascularisation [66–69]. Various studies found certain pore sizes were better suited for the development of various tissue and cell types [70–72]. For example Dehghani et al. describe that most suitable pore sizes for neovascularisation of a material is in the range of 5 μm, while larger pores between 20 μm and 125 μm are optimal for hepatocyte ingrowth and skin regeneration. In addition, pore sizes in the range of 100–350 μm are suitable for bone growth [70], but for the rapid vascularisation of tissue and survival of transplanted cells pores larger than 500 μm is required, although a separate study found that 250 μm provided the right balance of tissue infiltration and surface area for cellular attachment [71]. As a result of these requirements, when designing scaffolds, pore sizes need to be tailored to optimise the regeneration of such specific tissues.

Appropriate and controllable biodegradation rate is highly desirable and ideally the bulk mechanical properties, including the Young's modulus should match the surrounding tissue to enable the tissue to be remodelled, if biodegradable material is to be used to degrade at the rate of growth of invading tissue without undue foreign body reaction. Soft tissues possess highly variable Young's moduli; for example, muscle and liver tissues can possess low Young's moduli in the range of approximately 0.4 kPa to 2 kPa [73], while tissues such as breast adipose, kidney and prostate may possess moduli in the range of approximately 10 kPa to 70 kPa [74, 75]. As a result of this large variation, scaffolds targeted for specific tissue types need to possess Young's moduli to match that of the desired tissue.

Mechanical robustness of the hydrogel scaffold is also important in shielding the developing tissue from environmental forces. The mechanical strengths of scaffolds need to be tuned according to the environment, and the forces the scaffolds will experience due to the function of the tissue. On the other hand an appropriate surface is required to allow desired scaffold–cell interactions. For example, surface roughness can play a substantial role, whereby compared to smooth surfaces, surfaces with increased roughness can lead to improved cell attachment and biocompatibility [76].

To date many of the hydrogels used for soft tissue engineering applications have been too weak [53] and unable to maintain the space to enable tissue growth, or they have been too stiff resulting in unwanted foreign body reactions and detachment from host tissues [76]. There are however a number of areas where hydrogels have found application and they are discussed below.

5.5 Applications of Hydrogels for Tissue Regeneration

Hydrogels are highly versatile and can be synthesised using a variety of techniques. The resultant hydrogels can display the desired properties for scaffolds successfully while retaining tissue like properties. Due to these advantages, hydrogels have been studied for numerous tissue engineering applications with promising outcomes.

5.5.1 *Cell Encapsulation and Delivery*

Due to their simple fabrication and biocompatible nature, hydrogels have been utilised in the delivery of cells or tissue inducing substances. As a result of their permeable nature, hydrogels are able to provide protection and support to cells while allowing the diffusion of nutrients and metabolites [77]. The cell and hydrogel types can be matched according to the method of cell encapsulation that is required [41–43]. For example, oxidised alginate hydrogels have been used as a means to deliver adipogenic cells for adipose tissue engineering [44], while a variety of hydrogels produced from materials including collagen and chitosan were utilised for cardiac tissue engineering by transplanting cardiomyocytes encased in such hydrogels [45–47].

Rossi et al. have developed photopolymerisable hyaluronic acid hydrogels for the delivery of satellite and muscle progenitor cells for muscle tissue repair [78]. These hyaluronic acid based hydrogels were developed for in situ curing of the hydrogel–cell combination in vivo in the injury site. In situ photopolymerisation offers the advantage of facile delivery of cells in a hydrogel network that would be able to take the shape of the defect site prior to curing. This would in turn allow the regeneration of tissue to match the target tissue site. Application of the hyaluronic acid hydrogels in injured mice muscles showed muscle structure regeneration while providing improved function. Liu et al. on the other hand developed microbeads encased in an alginate and Arg–Gly–Asp (RGD) based hydrogel [79]. The microbeads produced from alginate and fibrin were designed as biodegradable carriers for human umbilical cord stem cells (hUCMSCs) that would be released while creating macropores within the hydrogel matrix. Hence, the alginate–RGD hydrogel would be able to act as a porous scaffold following microbead degradation to provide the support for the hUCMSCs and fill the injured tissue defect.

Trauma, disease and surgical procedures can lead to significant loss of adipose tissue necessitating reconstruction [76]. Adipose tissue engineering has involved the study of a variety of techniques for regenerative purposes. A method that has been investigated is the delivery of adipogenic cells via encapsulation with hydrogels. Hydrogels derived from collagen and alginate have been utilised for the fabrication of cell/hydrogel vehicles to promote the formation of fat tissue in the target area where loss of adipose tissue occurred [80, 81].

In addition, pancreatic islet cells, mesenchymal stem cells and tissue inducing substances such as various growth factors have been studied for delivery using hydrogel encapsulation [82–84]. The extensive application of hydrogels demonstrates their suitability as cell and substance vehicles for tissue engineering purposes.

5.5.2 *Hydrogels as Tissue Regeneration Substrates*

Tissue engineering entails the regeneration of tissues either directly in vivo or indirectly via in vitro growth and subsequent implantation in vivo Hydrogels have also been investigated as constructs to support regeneration of tissues both in vitro and in vivo. Hydrogels possess desirable properties that make them suitable for such applications.

In order to repair tissues that have undergone damage such as during myocardial infarction, grafts of regenerated tissue may be necessary. For example Giraud et al. developed skeletal muscle grafts for the treatment of infarcted cardiac tissue by regenerating myoblasts in a collagenous hydrogel in vitro [85]. Furthermore, Hosseini et al. engineered skeletal muscle-like structures on hydrogel substrates [86]. The methacrylated hydrogels presented microgrooves on their surface that allowed alignment of myofibres and ultimate formation of muscle sheets in vitro that could be utilised as grafts for reconstruction of damaged skeletal muscle tissue. On the other hand, regeneration of smooth muscle for intestinal and blood vessel tissue engineering have garnered interest via the use of hydrogels. Culture of smooth muscle cells in a fibrin hydrogel and their subsequent seeding onto chitosan/collagen scaffolds have been described to produce smooth muscle for intestinal tissue engineering applications [87]. Alternatively, aortic smooth muscle has been cultured via a layer-by-layer technique in microchannels with the use of alginate hydrogels as layering support. Smooth muscle tissue sheets were developed with the hydrogel layers in order to assist in the formation of aligned tissues, which is not observed when cells are simply encapsulated in a matrix [88].

Hydrogels have also found uses in corneal applications. The foremost reason behind corneal transplantation is the loss of function of corneal endothelial cells (CECs) [89, 90]. CECs are specialised, polygonally shaped cells that reside on the inner surface of the cornea, responsible for actively pumping fluids across the cornea to preserve corneal transparency [90]. Various factors can lead to the loss of CECs, such as aging, trauma and disease [89, 91], leading to blindness. We have previously produced a chitosan-PEG hydrogel film that supports the attachment and proliferation of CECs in vitro and demonstrated that the cultured cells maintain their native morphology [92]. In addition, we have demonstrated ex vivo that these hydrogel films possess excellent tensile properties that make them suitable for implantation purposes.

As mentioned previously, scaffolds need to possess appropriate interconnected pores to provide the required environment for uniform tissue development. A range of techniques have been exploited to produce porous scaffolds, including porogen leaching, gas foaming, thermally induced phase separation (TIPS) and electro-spinning [93–96]. Hydrogels also need to possess such porous structures in order to be successful as scaffolds. For example, Park et al. showed that porous PEG–PCL scaffolds prepared via a salt-leaching technique permit the formation of neocartilage within four weeks, when implanted in mice [63]. Also, we have previously demonstrated that biodegradable, salt-templated porous PEG hydrogels produced via epoxy-amine chemistry allowed the penetration of cellular and vascular tissue within two weeks in a rat model [65]. The PEG hydrogels were able to allow rapid vascularisation and tissue penetration within two weeks while providing the appropriate mechanical integrity to allow the proliferation of tissue.

5.5.3 *Complete Replacement of Tissues*

Hydrogels designed as scaffolds for the regeneration of tissues are generally tailored to biodegrade in order to be ultimately replaced by healthy regenerating tissue. In certain cases, it may not be necessary to regenerate the compromised tissue, but instead replace it with a synthetic alternative. Due to their high water content and network structures resembling the ECM, hydrogels have also found potential applications in the complete replacement of tissues. Such hydrogels are designed to be non-degradable and maintain their structure as permanent tissue substitute to provide basic functions of tissues. Certain tissues such as the cornea, ligaments and other load bearing tissues may potentially be replaced with hydrogels that can mimic their basic function [77]. Such hydrogel materials need to display the required function of the target tissue satisfactorily to be considered as a substitute.

For example, Gong et al. developed double network (DN) hydrogels that are extremely resistant to compression and tearing as potential replacements for load bearing tissues [53]. These hydrogels could withstand 25 MPa of shear force and were designed in consideration of the needs of load bearing tissues such as articular cartilage, tendons and ligaments. Other studies looked into the replacement of nucleus pulposus (NP), a natural gel present in the middle of invertebral discs designed to resist and distribute compressive forces [51]. Due to its composite nature, simple replacement of the NP with a homogenous material may not be sufficient; as such Strange et al. described the study of a multi-phase hydrogel to better replicate the non-homogenous behaviour of such tissues [51].

Other soft tissues such as the vitreous humour in the eye may need partial or complete replacement following vitreoretinal surgery or vitrectomy [92]. Various materials have been considered as replacement for the vitreous humour [97], which includes hydrogels. Due to the needs of the eye, proposed substitutes need to possess variety of functionalities such as biocompatibility and transparency. Due to the possibility of functionalisation and modification during synthesis, hydrogels are well suited. To this end, hydrogels based on poly(vinyl alcohol) and methyl acrylamidoglycolate methyl ether (MAGME) have been evaluated as potential replacements for vitreous humour, with favourable physico-chemical properties [97, 98].

Corneal transplantation is a procedure in which the diseased cornea of a patient is replaced by healthy donor tissue [89]. Various transplantation methods are available ranging from the replacement of the whole cornea to the replacement of the diseased cell layer only [99–102]. Certain patients are under high risk of graft failure due to previous corneal transplantation procedures, and to address this need, a synthetic commercial corneal substitute AlphaCor™ has been developed [103]. AlphaCor™ is a synthetic hydrogel produced from PHEMA that possess two phases, a central transparent region for optical needs and a porous peripheral region that allows integration of the synthetic cornea with the surrounding tissue. Clinical studies have shown favourable results with the implantation of AlphaCor™ demonstrating the potential, and suitability of hydrogels as replacements of tissue in vivo.

5.6 Summary

There are certain physico-chemical properties tissue engineering scaffolds need to possess in order to be successful in the regeneration of tissues. Hydrogels are hydrophilic networks that can be synthesised from various polymers of both natural and synthetic origin and can mimic the properties of natural tissues. As a result these desirable properties hydrogels of various origins have been investigated for applications in the delivery of cells, replacement, regeneration and repair of various tissue types in vitro and in vitro. The tailorability and functionality of hydrogels make them highly versatile and suitable for tissue engineering applications. As demonstrated by various studies that exploit their favourable characteristics, hydrogels continue to be one of the most attractive group of materials for both biomedical and tissue engineering purposes.

References

1. Langer R, Vacanti JP. Tissue engineering. *Science* 1993; 260:920–926.
2. Kaihara S, Vacanti JP. Tissue Engineering—toward new solutions for transplantation and reconstructive surgery. *Arch Surg* 1999; 134(11):1184–1188.
3. Freed LE, Vunjack-Novakovic G, Biron RJ, et al. Biodegradable polymer scaffolds for tissue engineering. *Biotechnol* 1994; 12(7):680–693.
4. Hutmacher DW. Scaffold design and fabrication technologies for engineering tissues—state of the art and future perspectives. *J Biomater Sci Polym Ed* 2001; 12(1):107–124.
5. Kasemo B, Biological surface science. *Surf Sci* 2002; 500:656–677.
6. Elbert DL, Hubbel JA. Surface treatments of polymers for biocompatibility. *Annu Rev Mater Sci* 1996; 26:365–394.
7. Ma Z, Mao Z, Gao C. Surface modification and property analysis of biomedical polymers used for tissue engineering. *Colloids Surf B* 2007; 60:137–157.
8. Anderson JM, Jones JA. Phenotypic dichomoties in the foreign body reaction. *Biomaterials* 2007; 28:5114–5120.
9. Brodbeck WG, Nakayama Y, Matsuda T, Colton E, Ziats NP, Anderson JM. Biomaterial surface chemistry dictates adherent monocyte/macrophage cytokine expression in vitro. *Cytokine* 2002; 18(6):311-319.
10. Keselowsky BG, Bridges AW, Burns KL, et al. Role of plasma fibronectin in the foreign body response to biomaterials. *Biomaterials* 2007; 28:3626–3631.
11. Dinnes DLM, Santerre JP, Labow RS. Influence of biodegradable and non-biodegradable material surfaces on the differentiation of human monocyte-derived macrophages. *Differentiation* 2008; 76:232–244.
12. Guan J, Stankus JJ, Wagner WR. Biodegradable elastomeric scaffolds with basic fibroblast growth factor release. *J Control Release* 2007; 120:70–78.
13. Bramfeldt H, Sabra G, Centis V, Vermette P. Scaffold vascularization: A challenge for three-dimensional tissue engineering. *Curr Med Chem* 2010; 17:3944–3967.
14. Liu X, Holzwarth JM, Ma PX. Functionalized synthetic biodegradable polymer scaffolds for tissue engineering. *Macromol Biosci* 2012; 12:911–919.

15. Hoffman AS. Hydrogels for biomedical applications. *Anns NY Acad Sci* 2001; 944:62–73.
16. Kawazoe N, Inoue C, Tateishi T, Chen G. A cell leakproof PLGA-collagen hybrid scaffold for cartilage tissue engineering. *Biotechnol Prog* 2010; 26(3):819–826.
17. Valente JFA, Valente TAM, Alves P, Ferreira P, Silva A, Correia IJ. Alginate based scaffolds for bone tissue engineering. *Mat Sci Eng C* 2012; 32:2596–2603.
18. Wen P, Gao J, Zhang Y, et al. Fabrication of chitosan scaffolds with tunable porous orientation structure for tissue engineering. *J Biomater Sci Polym Ed* 2011; 22:19–40.
19. Gervaso F, Scalera F, Padmanabhan SK, Sannino A, Licciulli A. High-performance hydroxyapatite scaffolds for bone tissue engineering applications. *Int J Appl Ceram Technol* 2012; 9(3):597–516.
20. Kim S, Healy KE. Synthesis and characterisation of injectable poly(N-isopropylacrylamide-co-acyrlic acid) hydrogels with proteolytically degradable cross-links. *Biomacromolecules* 2003; 4:1214–1223.
21. Adds PJ, Hunt CJ, Dart JKG. Amniotic membrane grafts, "fresh" or "frozen"? A clinical and in vitro comparison. *Br J Ophthalmol* 2001; 85:905–907.
22. Angelova N, Hunkeler D. Rationalising the design of polymeric biomaterials. *Trends Biotechnol* 1999; 17:409–421.
23. Zhu H, Ji J, Shen J. Surface engineering of poly(DL-lactic acid) by entrapment of biomacromolecules. *Macromol Rapid Commun* 2002; 23:819–823.
24. Ko HF, Sfeir C, Kumta PN. Novel synthesis strategies for natural polymer and composite biomaterials as potential scaffolds for tissue engineering. *Phil Trans R Soc A* 2010; 368:1981–1997.
25. Liang Y, Liu W, Han B, et al. Fabrication and characters of a corneal endothelial cells scaffold based on chitosan. *J Mater Sci Mater Med* 2011; 22:175–183.
26. Lu DR, Xiao CM, Xu SJ. Starch-based completely biodegradable polymer materials. *Express Polym Lett* 2009; 3(6):366–375.
27. Sachlos E, Czerbuszka JT. Making tissue engineering scaffolds work: Review on the application of solid freeform fabrication technology to the production of tissue engineering scaffolds. *Eur Cell Mater* 2003; 5:29–40.
28. Sadr N, Pippenger BE, Scherberich A, et al. Enhancing the biological performance of synthetic polymeric materials by decoration with

engineered, decellularized extracellular matrix. *Biomaterials* 2012; 33:5085–5093.

29. Mistry AS, Cheng SH, Yeh T, Christenson E, Jansen JA, Mikos A. Fabrication and in vitro degradation of porous fumarate-based polymer/alumoxane nanocomposite scaffolds for bone tissue engineering. *J Biomed Mater Res A* 2009; 89(1):68–79.
30. Svobodová J, Rypáček F. Polyglutamate copolymers as a tissue-engineering platform: Polymer scaffold modification through aminolysis of poly(γ-benzyl-l-glutamate-co-2,2,2-γ-trichlorethyl-l-glutamate). *Eur Polym J* 2012; 48(1):183–190.
31. Jiang X, Yu F, Wang Z, et al. Fabrication and characterization of waterborne biodegradable polyurethanes 3-dimensional porous scaffolds for vascular tissue engineering. *J Biomater Sci Polym Ed* 2010; 21(12):1637–1652.
32. Park S, Park D, Shin J, et al. Scaffolds for bone tissue engineering fabricated from two different materials by the rapid prototyping technique: PCL versus PLGA. *J Mater Sci Mater Med* 2012; 23(11):2671–2678.
33. Kawazoe N, Inoue C, Tateishi T, Chen G. A cell leakproof PLGA-collagen hybrid scaffold for cartilage tissue engineering. *Biotechnol Prog* 2010; 26(3):819–826.
34. Marler JJ, Upton J, Langer R, Vacanti JP. Transplantation of cells in matrices for tissue regeneration. *Adv Drug Deliv Rev* 1998; 33:165–182.
35. Lee JW, Gardella JA. Surface perspectives in the biomedical applications of poly(α-hydroxy acids) and their associate copolymers. *Anal Bioanal Chem* 2002; 373:526–537.
36. Drury JL, Mooney DJ. Hydrogels for tissue engineering: scaffold design variables and applications. *Biomaterials* 2003; 24:4337–4351.
37. Hoffman AS. Hydrogels for biomedical applications. *Adv Drug Deliv Rev* 2012; 64:18–23.
38. Hoare TR, Kohane DS. Hydrogels in drug delivery: Progress and challenges. *Polymer* 2008; 49:1993–2007.
39. Kopecek J, Yang J. Hydrogels as smart biomaterials. *Polymer Int* 2007; 56:1078–1098.
40. Lee KY, Mooney DJ. Hydrogels for tissue engineering. *Chem Rev* 2001; 101(7):1869–1877.
41. Jen AC, Wake MC, Mikos AG. Hydrogels for cell immobilisation. *Biotechnol Bioeng* 1996; 50(4):357–364.

42. Alsberg E, Anderson KW, Albeiruti A, Franceschi RT, Mooney DJ. Cell-interactive alginate hydrogels for bone tissue engineering. *J Dent Res* 2001; 80(11):2025–2029.
43. De Chalain T, Phillips JH, Hinek A. Bioengineering of elastic cartilage with aggregated porcine and human auricular chondrocytes and hydrogels containing alginate, collagen and K-elastin, *J Biomed Mater Res A* 1999; 44(3):280–288.
44. Kim W, Mooney D, Arany P, et al. Adipose tissue engineering using injectable, oxidized alginate hydrogels. *Tissue Eng A* 2012; 18(7–8):737–743.
45. Li Z, Guan J. Hydrogels for cardiac tissue engineering. *Polymers* 2011; 3(2):740–761.
46. Reis L, Chiu L, Liang Y, Hyunh K, Momen A, Radisic M. A peptide-modified chitosan-collagen hydrogel for cardiac cell culture and delivery. *Acta Biomaterialia* 2012; 8(3):1022–1036.
47. Chiu L, Janic K, Radisic M. Engineering of oriented myocardium on three-dimensional micropatterned collagen-chitosan hydrogel. *Int J Artif Organs* 2012; 35(4):237–250.
48. Guarino V, Gloria A, Raucci M, Ambrosio L. Hydrogel-based platforms for the regeneration of osteochondral tissue and intervertebral disc. *Polymers* 2012; 4(3):1590–1612.
49. Li F, Ba QJ, Niu SM, et al. In-situ forming biodegradable glycol chitosan-based hydrogels: Synthesis, characterization, and chondrocyte culture. *Mater Sci Eng C Mater Biol Appl* 2012; 32(7):2017–2025.
50. Lind M, Larsen A, Clausen C, Osther K, Everland H. Cartilage repair with chondrocytes in fibrin hydrogel and MPEG polylactide scaffold: An in vivo study in goats. *Knee Surg Sport Tr A* 2008; 16(7):690–698.
51. Strange D, Oyen M. Composite hydrogels for nucleus pulposus tissue engineering. *J Mech Behav Biomed* 2012; 11:16–26.
52. Hu JG, Chen B, Guo F, et al. Injectable silk fibroin/polyurethane composite hydrogel for nucleus pulposus replacement. *J Mater Sci Mater Med* 2012; 23(3):711–722.
53. Gong JP, Katsuyama Y, Kurokawa T, Osada Y. Double network hydrogels with extremely high mechanical strength. *Adv Mater* 2003; 15(14):1155–1158.
54. Merchant RE, Zhu J. Design properties of hydrogel tissue engineering scaffolds. *Exp Rev Med Dev* 2011; 8(5):607–626.

55. Ronda L, Bruno S, Abbruzzetti S, Viappiani C, Bettati S. Ligand reactivity and allosteric regulation of haemoglobin based oxygen carriers. *Biochim Biophys Acta* 2008; 1784:1365–1377.

56. Bailon P, Berhtold W. Polyethylene glycol-conjugated pharmaceutical proteins. *Pharm Sci Technol Today* 1998; 1(8):352–356.

57. Kim DN, Lee W, Koh WG. Preparation of protein microarrays on non-fouling and hydrated poly(ethylene glycol) hydrogel substrates using photochemical surface modification. *J Chem Technol Biotechnol* 2009; 84:279–284.

58. Quirk RA, Davies MC, Tendler SJB, Chan WC, Shakesheff KM. Controlling biological interactions with poly(lactic acid) by surface entrapment modification. *Langmuir* 2001; 17:2817–2820.

59. Shen M, Pan YV, Wagner MS, et al. Inhibition of monocyte adhesion and fibrinogen adsorption on glow discharge plasma deposited tetraethylene glycol dimethyl ether. *J Biomat Sci Polym Ed* 2001; 12(9):961–978.

60. Dalton PD, Hostert C, Albrecht K, Moeller M, Groll J. Structure and properties of urea-crosslinked star poly(ethylene oxide)-ran-(proplyene oxide) hydrogels. *Macromol Biosci* 2008; 8:923–931.

61. Tan H, DeFail AJ, Rubin JP, Chu CR, Marra KG. Novel multiarm PEG-based hydrogels for tissue engineering. *J Biomed Res A* 2010; 92A(3):979–987.

62. Han DK, Park KD, Hubbel JA, Kim YH. Surface characteristics and biocompatibility of lactide-based poly(ethylene glycol) scaffolds for tissue engineering. *J Biomat Sci Polym E* 1998; 9(7):667–680.

63. Park JS, Woo DG, Sun BK, et al. In vitro and in vivo test of PEG/PCL-based hydrogel scaffold for cell delivery application. *J Control Release* 2007; 124(1–2):51–59.

64. Park CH, Hong YJ, Park K, Han DK. Peptide-grafted lactide-based poly(ethylene glycol) porous scaffolds for specific cell adhesion. *Macromol Res* 2010; 18(5):526–532.

65. Hamid ZAA, Blencowe A, Ozcelik B, et al. Epoxy-amine synthesised hydrogel scaffolds for soft-tissue engineering. *Biomaterials* 2010; 31:6454–6467.

66. Chiu YC, Cheng MH, Engel H, et al. The role of pore size on vascularization and tissue remodelling in PEG hydrogels. *Biomaterials* 2011; 32:6045–6051.

67. Ko YG, Oh HH, Kawazoe N, Tateishi T, Chen G. Preparation of open porous hyaluronic acid scaffolds for tissue engineering using the ice

particulate template method. *J Biomater Sci Polym Ed* 2011; 22:123–138.

68. Sukmana I. Bioactive polymer scaffold for fabrication of vascularized engineering tissue. *J Artif Organs* 2012; 15:215–224.
69. Sicchieri LG, Crippa GE, de Oliveira PT, Belot MM, Rosa AL. Pore size regulates cell and tissue interactions with PLGA-CaP scaffolds used for bone engineering. *J Tissue Eng Regen M* 2012; 6(2):155–162.
70. Dehghani F, Annabi N. Engineering porous scaffolds using gas-based techniques. *Curr Opin Biotechnol* 2011; 22:661–666.
71. Yamamoto M, Tabata Y, Kawasaki H, Ikada Y. Promotion of fibrovascular tissue ingrowth into porous sponges by basic fibroblast growth factor. *J Mater Sci Mater Med* 2000; 11(4):213–218.
72. Yang SF, Leong KF, Du ZH, Chua CK. The design of scaffolds for use in tissue engineering Part I: Traditional factors. *Tissue Eng* 2001; 7(6):679–689.
73. Chen E, Novakofski J, Jenkins W, OBrien W. Young's modulus measurements of soft tissues with application to elasticity imaging. *IEEE Trans Ultrason Ferroelectr Freq Contr* 1996; 43(1):191–194.
74. Krouskop TA, Wheeler TM, Kallel F, Garra BS, Hall T. Elastic moduli of breast and prostate tissues under compression. *Ultrason Imaging* 1998; 20:260–274.
75. Erkamp RQ, Wiggins P, Skovoroda AR, Emelianov SY, O'Donnell M. Measuring the elastic modulus of small tissue samples. *Ultrason Imaging* 1998; 20(1):17–28.
76. Hakeam G, Eid K, Sharaf M, Badr Y, Abbass M, Solouma N. Laser surface modification of poly(ε-caprolactone) scaffold for artificial skin applications, *Am J Biomed Sci* 2013; 5(1):1–13.
77. Slaughter BV, Khurshid SS, Fisher OZ, Khademhosseini A, Peppas NA. Hydrogels in regenerative medicine. *Adv Mater* 2009; 21:3307–3329.
78. Rossi CA, Flaibani M, Blaauw B, et al. In vivo tissue engineering of functional skeletal muscle by freshly isolated satellite cells embedded in a photopolymerizable hydrogel. *FASEB J* 2011; 25:2296–2304.
79. Liu J, Zhou H, Weir MD, Xu HHK, Chen Q, Trotman CA. Fast-degradable microbeads encapsulating human umbilical cord stem cells in alginate for muscle tissue engineering. *Tissue Eng A* 2012; 18(21–22):2303–2314.
80. Yao R, Zhang RJ, Lin F, Luan J. Injectable cell/hydrogel microspheres induce the formation of fat lobule-like microtissues and vascularized adipose tissue regeneration. *Biofabrication* 2012; 4:1–10.

81. Galateanu B, Dimonie D, Vasile E, Nae S, Cimpean A, Costache M. Layer-shaped alginate hydrogels enhance the biological performance of human adipose-derived stem cells. *BMC Biotechnol* 2012; 12:35–48.
82. Davis NE, Beenken-Rothkopf LN, Mirsoian A, et al. Enhanced function of pancreatic islets co-encapsulated with ECM proteins and mesenchymal stromal cells in a silk hydrogel. *Biomaterials* 2012; 33(28):6691–6697.
83. Lee JY, Shin JM, Yeum CE, Chae GT, Chun MH, Oh SJ. Intravitreal delivery of mesenchymal stem cells loaded onto hydrogel affects the regulatory expression of endogenous NGF and BDNF in ischemic rat retina. *J Tissue Eng Regen M* 2012; 9(5):249–258.
84. Salimath AS, Phelps EA, Boopathy AV, et al. Dual delivery of hepatocyte and vascular endothelial growth factors via a protease-degradable hydrogel improves cardiac function in rats. *PLoS One* 2012; 7:1–12.
85. Giraud MN, Ayuni E, Cook S, Siepe M, Carrel TP, Tevaearai HT. Hydrogel-based engineered skeletal muscle grafts normalize heart function early after myocardial infarction. *Artif Organs* 2008; 32(9):692–700.
86. Hosseini V, Ahadian S, Ostrovidov S, et al. Engineered contractile skeletal muscle tissue on a microgrooved methacrylated gelatin substrate. *Tissue Eng A* 2012; 18(23–24):2453–2465.
87. Zakhem E, Raghavan S, Gilmont RR, Bitar KN. Chitosan-based scaffolds for the support of smooth muscle constructs in intestinal tissue engineering. *Biomaterials* 2012; 33:4810–4817.
88. Rayatpisheh S, Poon YF, Cao Y, Feng J, Chan V, Chan-Park MB. Aligned 3D human aortic smooth muscle tissue via layer by layer technique inside microchannels with novel combination of collagen and oxidized alginate hydrogel. *J Biomed Mater Res A* 2011; 98A:235–244.
89. Engelmann K, Bednarz J, Valtnik M. Prospects for endothelial transplantation. *Exp Eye Res* 2004; 78:573–578.
90. Peh GSL, Beuerman RW, Colman A, Tan DT, Mehta JS. Human corneal endothelial cell expansion for corneal endothelium transplantation: An Overview. *Transplantation* 2011; 91(8):811–819.
91. Joyce NC. Proliferative capacity of the corneal endothelium. *Prog Retin Eye Res* 2003; 22:359–389.
92. Ozcelik B, Brown K, Blencowe A, Daniell M, Stevens GW, Qiao GG. Ultrathin chitosan–poly(ethylene glycol) hydrogel films for corneal tissue engineering. *Acta Biomaterialia* 2013, http://dx.doi.org/10.1016/j.actbio.2013.01.020

93. Gong XH, Tang CY, Zhang YG, Wong Ct, Wu SP, Liu JN. Fabrication of graded macroporous poly(lactic acid) scaffold by a progressive solvent casting/porogen leaching approach. *J Appl Polym Sci* 2012; 125:571–577.
94. Huang YY, Wang DY, Chang LL, Yang YC. Fabricating microparticles/nanofibers composite and nanofiber scaffold with controllable pre size by rotating multichannel electrospinning. *J Biomater Sci Polym Ed* 2010; 21:1503–1514.
95. Pavia FC, La Carrubba V, Brucato V. Morphology and thermal properties of foams prepared via thermally induced phase separation based on polylactic acid blends. *J Cell Plast* 2012; 48(5):399–407.
96. Dehghani F, Annabi N. Engineering porous scaffolds using gas-based techniques. *Curr Opin Biotechnol* 2011; 22:661–666.
97. Cavalieri F, Miano F, D'Antona P, Paradossi G. Study of gelling behavior of poly(vinyl alcohol)-methacrylate for potential utilizations in tissue replacement and drug delivery. *Biomacromolecules* 2004; 5:2439–2446.
98. Chirila TV, Constable IJ, Hong Y, et al. Synthetic hydrogel as an artificial vitreous body—A one year animal study on its effects on the retina. *Cell Mater* 1995; 5:83–96.
99. Armitage WJ, Tullo AB, Larkin DFP. The first successful full-thickness corneal transplant: A commentary on Eduard Zirm's landmark paper of 1906. *Br J Ophthalmol* 2006; 90:1222–1223.
100. Melles GRJ, Eggink F, Lander F, et al. A surgical technique for posterior lamellar keratoplasty. *Cornea* 1998; 17(6):618–626.
101. Melles GRJ, Ong TS, Ververs B, van der Wees J. Descemet membrane endothelial keratoplasty. *Cornea* 2006; 25(8):987–990.
102. Dapena I, Ham L, Melles GRJ. Endothelial keratoplasty: DSEK/DSAEK or DMEK—the thinner the better? *Curr Opin Ophthalmol* 2009; 20:299–307.
103. Hicks CR, Crawford GJ, Lou X, et al Corneal replacement using a synthetic hydrogel cornea, AlphaCor^{TM}: device, preliminary outcomes and complications. *Eye* 2003; 17(3):385–392.

Chapter 6

Polyethylene Glycol Gel for Orthopaedic Technologies

Masanori Kobayashi
Biomedical Engineering Department, Daido University, 10-3 Takiharu-cho, Minami-ku, Nagoya, 536-4876 Japan
mkoba@daido-it.ac.jp

In this article, some basic properties of polyethylene glycol (PEG) gel will be briefly introduced, together with the clinical advantages as well as the effects observed during the study of this polymer for biomedical purposes. Although the practical application of PEG to orthopaedic field is still restricted, this hydrate material is a potential alternative biopolymers for orthopaedics surgery, taking into account the unique characteristics.

6.1 Introduction

Orthopaedic surgery or orthopaedics is the branch of surgery concerned with conditions involving the musculoskeletal system. In this field, many biomaterials and prosthesis implants such as

Hydrated Materials: Applications in Biomedicine and the Environment
Edited by Yoshitaka Nakanishi

ISBN 978-981-4463-22-5 (Hardcover), 978-981-4463-23-2 (eBook)
www.panstanford.com

artificial joints, artificial bone, and instrumentation for bone fracture have been developed and used clinically for the long time [1, 2].

As for hydrate material and hydrogel, however, the clinical orthopaedic applications are very restricted because of their low mechanical strength and complicated characteristics. In near future, new hydrate biomaterials with new characteristic function will be developed and utilised in clinical application including the scaffold for tissue engineering in the future as a new method.

In this chapter, the author will overview a series of findings discovered so far regarding the clinical applications of this typical hydrate material, polyethylene glycol (PEG), as a treatment for the joint disease in the orthopaedic surgery.

6.2 Polyethylene Glycol

6.2.1 *The Basic Characteristics Properties of PEG*

PEG is the polymer represents following chemical formula HO–$(CH_2CH_2OH)_n$–H, which refers to a chemical compound composed of repeating ethylene glycol units.

PEG has long been manufactured industrially and utilised in many applications such as non-ionic surfactants, lubricants, and an intermediate for urethane composition, adhesives, and cosmetics. PEG is non-toxic and is also used for bio-related applications such as pharmaceutical formulation, aqueous two-phase partition, precipitant for plasmid DNA isolation, protein crystallisation, and cell fusion.

Among water-soluble polymers, PEG has the following important characteristics. Firstly, PEG can form a good interaction between a polymer and solvent. This means that PEG is completely miscible in water, owing to the hydrogen bonding between water molecules and ether oxygen in the PEG chain. PEG has one of the largest second virial coefficients among hydrophilic polymers, which means that it adopts a well-expanded conformation in water. Secondly, PEG also has a small mobility factor value, which means high mobility in aqueous media. Thus, PEG has a high water compatibility, large exclusion volume, and extremely high flexibility (Fig. 6.1).

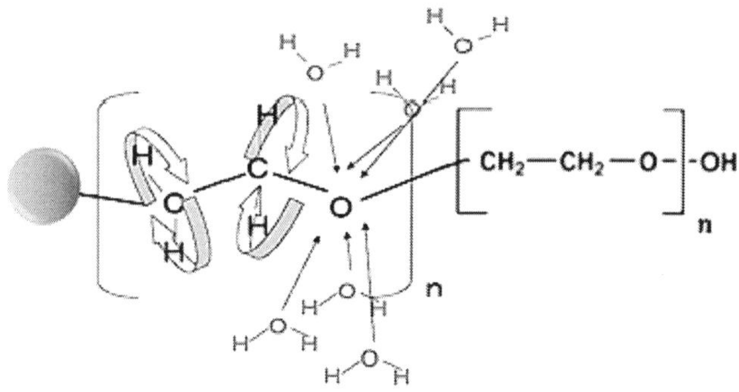

Figure 6.1 The PEG molecular structure.

With the OH groups at the ends of the PEG molecules, all reactions typical for alcohols are possible, first of all esters buildings among others as carbonates and carbamates formation. Thus, replacing the free end of PEG molecules to another organic group, PEG is able to have an important role in the high-performance of biological functions; this advantageous hydrate material has attracted growing interest as a biomedical application such as bio-separations, bio-imaging, bio-chip and drug mediator [3, 4].

On the other hand, as not a functional materials but a structural material, PEG hydrogels has been of great interest in tissue engineering and biomaterials field because of their established biocompatibility, high permeability, and tuneable material properties. But, the rational design of PEG hydrogel properties has been inhibited by the interdependence of key material properties such as modulus and mesh size, some studies have tried to achieve the appropriate mechanical properties for scaffold or artificial prosthesis [5, 6].

6.2.2 *The Applications for Bio-Medicine*

From these perspectives, PEG has begun to have an important role in the development of biomedical application. Especially, the studies regarding the bio-interfaces and drug delivery system (DDS) have been aggressively advanced.

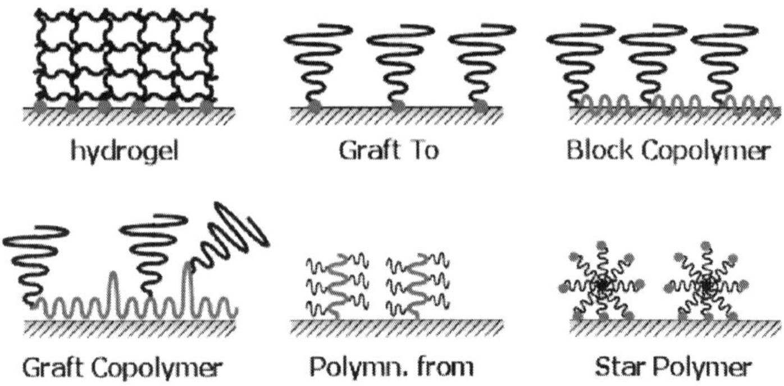

Figure 6.2 The schema of surface modifications achieved using PEG derivatives. Reprinted with permission from Ref. [3].

6.2.2.1 Bio-interface

As mentioned above, PEG has an important role in the development of bio-interfaces. This is especially true regarding the versatile techniques for surface coating using PEG that have been developed since 1980s to improve blood and biocompatibility. Figure 6.2 summarises several methods for the immobilisation of PEG on substrate surfaces, they are PEG gels, the physical and chemical immobilisation of PEG (so-called grafting to method), the adsorption of block and graft copolymers, polymerisation from the surface (the so-called grafting-from method), the immobilisation of star-shaped polymers and micelles and other methods.

Recently, the technique to construct PEG tethered chains on the surfaces, that is grafting technique, has been improved by inducing a specific interaction between the polymer and the surface, hydrophobic interaction, electrostatic interaction or covalent conjugation [7]. By these techniques, the strategy for more active, sensitive and selective functional bio-interface could be employed for the preparation of PEG polymer.

6.2.2.2 Drug delivery system

Novel controlled DDS are designed to deliver drugs at predetermined rates for predefined periods at the target organ, which could be used to overcome the shortcomings of conventional drug formulations, therefore could diminish the side effects and improve the life quality of the patients. Thus, a suitable controlled DDS is extremely important for chemotherapy.

Hydrogels are a special class of macromolecules, which could absorb much water while maintaining their integrity in water. Over the past decades, the stimuli-sensitive hydrogel has attracted increasing attention owing to their responsiveness to the environmental stimulus, including chemical substances and changes in temperature, pH, or electric field. The biodegradable thermosensitive physical crosslinked hydrogels have been extensively studied due to their great biodegradability, biocompatibility, and responsiveness to temperature [8, 9].

Among these hydrogels, PEG gel is the most frequently and widely used. Along with its biocompatibility, other special characteristics contribute to the wide application of PEG. When PEG is conjugated to hydrophobic molecules, it adds hydrophilicity and increases the solubility of the conjugate. Furthermore, the large hydrodynamic volume of PEG can protect the conjugate from adhesion, aggregation, and enzymatic attack under biological conditions. Recently, some studies have made efforts to introduce selective biodegradability into PEG. The boundaries of PEG application could be further extended by biodegradability in response to the specific signals such as increase in temperature or pH. At present, PEG has been developed and studied in great depth to improve the curative effect of drugs.

In addition to these characteristics, some kinds of PEGs are able to react at one end of the molecule. This PEG conjugated to peculiar proteins and other organic molecules are developed as anticancer drugs, have attracted researcher's attention as useful material for DDS [10, 11].

6.2.3 *The Applications for Orthopaedic Surgery*

In orthopaedics field, the PEG gel has been expected as biosensor, DDS application, and scaffold material for tissue engineering.

Except these common applications such as applications, advantage of the mechanical rheological characteristics as a hydrated material of PEG has a potential to lead to a new medical treatment for the orthopaedics surgery, particularly in the field of joint disease.

The main component of synovial joint, articular cartilage is originally a hydrated gel, including synovial fluid as a sol, and chronic joint disease was caused by the disorder of these hydrate materials and lubricating function.

Although total knee arthroplasty (TKA) is a representative surgical treatment of this disease, it is associated with clinical problems concerning durability owing to wear of ultra-high-molecular-weight polyethylene (UHMWPE) components [12, 13].

These current problems are under the strategy by new technology and innovation, on occasion, the particular characteristics of PEG hydrate materials might have a potential to resolve the piece of these problems.

6.3 Background of Osteoarthritis (OA)

OA, the most common form of arthritis, is a chronic disease characterised by the slow degradation of cartilage, pain, and increasing disability. The disease can have an impact on several aspects of patient's life, including functional and activity of daily life, relationships, economic status, body image, and emotional well-being.

OA occurrence has a frequency in all of joints; above all, this introductory section summarises the presentations regarding the OA of knee joint, to which the PEG gel for a medical treatment is easily able to apply as an artificial articular cartilage, visco-supplementation for intra-articular injection.

6.3.1 *OA of the Knee Joint*

Joint articular cartilage and subchondral bone are the sites of major abnormalities in OA process. It should be noted that two primary pathologic responses are observed. One response is characterised by wear and structural break down of articular cartilages that proceed to development of focal erosions, diffuse area of the cartilage surface, and the appearance of gross ulceration. A second pathological response is characterised by proliferation of new bone

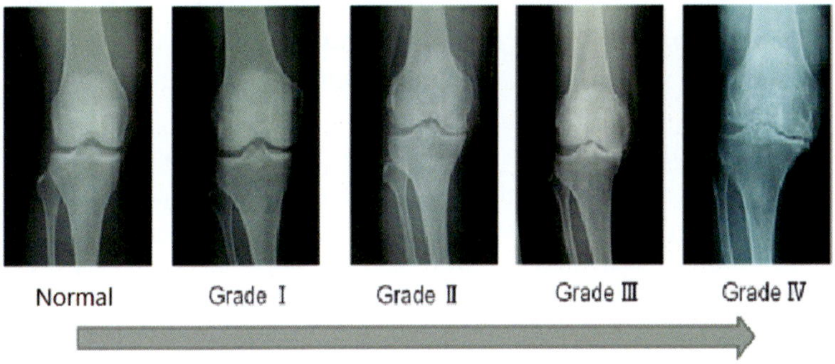

Figure 6.3 The radiographic progression of knee joint with OA. OA is classified into five stage or grade according to the progression.

and cartilage at the joint periphery that leads to osteochondrophyte spur, structural loss, bone formation and deformity. Pain, usually with activity, is virtually always a presenting complain of a patient with OA of the knee. Associated but less troublesome complains include stiffness, swelling in the knee and the restriction of rage of motion (ROM) of knee joint [14].

In the majority of the OA patients, there is no specific known underlying reason for the development of OA and the resulting deformity. However, of all the joints with OA, the knee joint best illustrates the contribution of biomechanics and biotribology factors to the development of OA and its progression. The primary concept involved at the knee is the interaction of increased loading stress and the response of the musculoskeletal system to this stress. An understanding of this concept is imperative in understanding OA of the knee joint and its management.

Figure 6.3 shows the X-ray photographs of each stages of OA progress in knee joint. The pathological appearances, narrowing of the joint space, osteophytes and bone deformity are observed with progression of OA.

6.3.2 *Conservative Treatment and Intra-Articular Injection of Hyaluronic Acid*

Although the OA of the knee is the most common of various articular disease, the mechanism of OA occurrence and progress has been still unclear, therefore, the treatment of OA of knee joint varies depending on the severity of symptoms, structural abnormalities present, the patient's age, chief complain and concomitant medical problems.

Current therapies are drug therapy, physical therapy, muscle exercise, therapy and rehabilitation. The goal of most patients is the relief of pain and localised stiffness; in addition, the prevention of deformity and associated limitation of motion.

Drug therapy is an important mainstay in the treatment of OA, analgesic and anti-inflammatory medication are often used. Although many patients can be effectively managed for long period, there are no specific agents for use in the treatment of OA that will prevent, retard, or reverse this disease at present. Therefore, some progressed OA patient with severe pain and dysfunction may need operative treatment.

As other treatment of OA knee joint, recently intra-articular injection method of high molecular weight hyaluronic acid (HA) has more widely accepted for releasing the pain. HA is responsible for the viscoelastic properties of synovial fluid, highviscos fluid. Its mechanism of action include two types, one is the biomechanics system, the enhancement of articular lubrication and fluid viscosity, another is the biological and biochemical system, the inhibition of inflammatory agent such as PGE2, NO, the suppression of proteoglycan from cartilage matrix, etc. [15–17].

6.3.3 *Total Knee Joint Arthroplasty (TKA)*

Orthopaedic procedures are important in the management of OA and should not be reserve only for late severe disease. TKA is the procedure of choice for OA associated with severe deformity. TKA represent advances that provide a quantum improvement in the overall quality of life desired by any given patient, with marked relief of pain and improvement in limitation of motion.

In prosthesis of knee joint, Co–Cr alloy is used as the femoral component and sliding surface, UHMWPE is used in the faced sliding surface of tibia components, the Co–Cr alloy or titanium alloy is utilised in the tibial tray underlying tibia (Fig. 6.4).

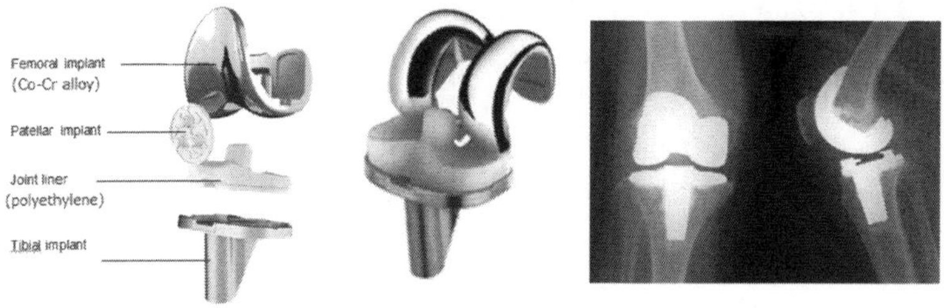

Figure 6.4 Artificial knee joint prosthesis.

Long-term follow-up reports suggested that knee arthroplasty is successful as a standard surgical treatment for OA. However, at the same time, long follow-up shows significant complication related to the durability of prosthesis. This problem of durability is mainly due to the wear of polyethylene (UHMWPE) of tibial component and following with the loosening of the prosthesis, and prosthesis fracture (Fig. 6.5).

In research field, this wear problem of UHMWPE has resulted in the development of biomaterial and innovative design towards reducing the complication and failure rate of the artificial joint. The cross-linked UHMWPE has been already identified and utilised as a superior material to polyethylene, many various improved implant design have been also proposed for reducing complication.

Furthermore, various studies regarding a new method for strengthening and fabrication of novel wear-resistant material, and 3D simulation and engineering of surgical techniques have

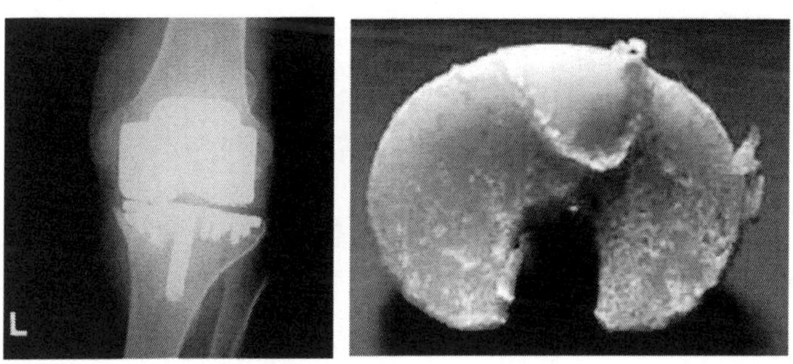

Figure 6.5 The wear of UHMWPE and aseptic loosening and osteolysis.

been studied in order to overcome this problem. Early results are encouraging, but further longterm outcome should be reported to evaluate the value [18, 19].

6.4 Development of Intra-Articular Artificial Lubricant Using PEG

According to the pathophysiology of OA of knee joint, OA is characterised by a slow degradation of cartilage over several years. In normal cartilage, a delicate balance exists between matrix synthesis and degradation; however, OA cartilage degradation exceeds synthesis or regeneration. The balance is affected and regulated by several factor such as age, weight etc. Considering that the biomechanical stress also belong to these factor, it would be highly effective for the medication and prevention of OA to improve the biomechanical and tribological circumstances for cartilage in knee joint by appropriate lubricant.

The concept of intra-articular injection of the HA for OA is also reasonable in the respects to this theory; however, the HA is easily degraded in the articular joint according to recent studies. Therefore new materials with excellent biocompatibility, durability, rheology and lubricative function are desired instead of the HA. The development of new intra-articular lubricant is an attractive theme for medical engineer, PEG sol as an artificial lubricant has been synthesised for medical treatment for OA knee.

The wear problem of UHMWPE in survival of TKA is also due to the same mechanical and tribological stress condition. An artificial lubricant development would be useful for the TKA longevity. This section introduces our work concerning PEG lubricant [20, 21].

6.4.1 *The Fabrication and Characteristics of PEG Lubricant*

For the artificial lubricant, PEG (molecular weight = 2 million) powder was prepared, and dissolved in distilled water, heated, and synthesised to 6 wt.% PEG hydrate sol material in Fig. 6.6.

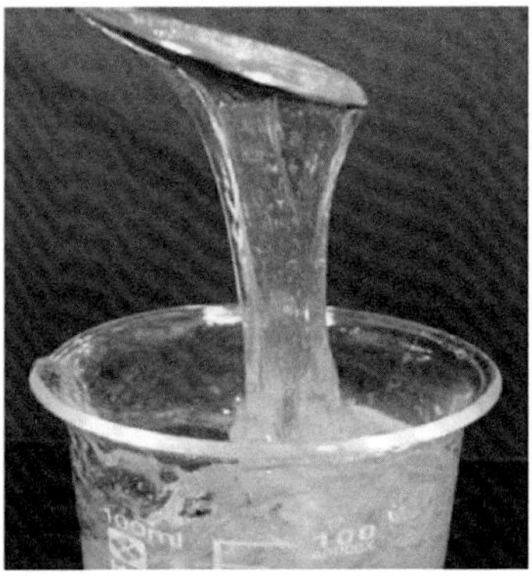

Figure 6.6 PEG lubricant sample (PEG 6 wt.%).

This water glycol hydraulic fluid has a three-dimensional network structure with H_2O molecules with high viscoelastic properties.

6.4.2 *Viscosity of PEG Lubricant*

The measured viscosity of this PEG lubricant and human synovial fluid is shown and compared in Fig. 6.7. The viscosity of PEG lubricant exhibits high value (about 280 dPa·stp) as compared with that of synovial fluid, and shows a non-Newtonian fluid changes depending on the shear rate.

6.4.3 *In Vivo Trial as Intra-Articular Lubricants for OA of the Knee*

Prior to the experiment intra-articular injections of PEG, the knee OA model rabbits were prepared by surgical procedure of the cartilage defect in the femoral condyle and meniscectomy and postoperative three months progress. As shown in Fig. 6.8, the knee joint of this experimental rabbits exhibit the early OA appearance such as progressive cartilage wear of the tibia and femoral.

While PEG lubricant was injected into one knee joint once a month for three months, another side as a control was kept under

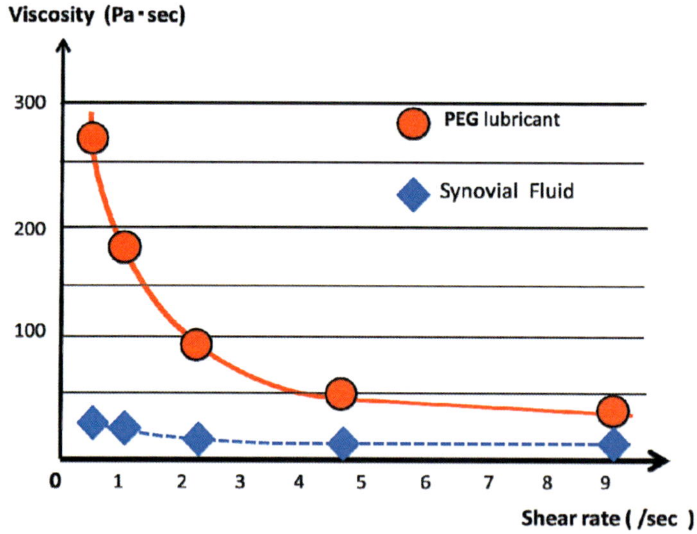

Figure 6.7 Viscosity curve of lubricants (PEG lubricant and synovial fluid).

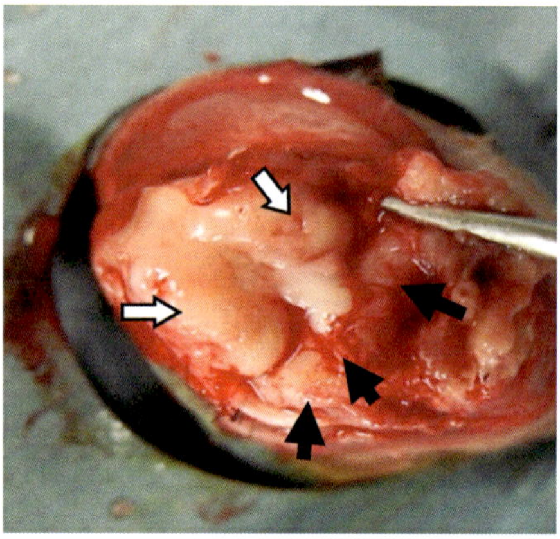

Figure 6.8 Appearance of OA model knee joint of rabbits.

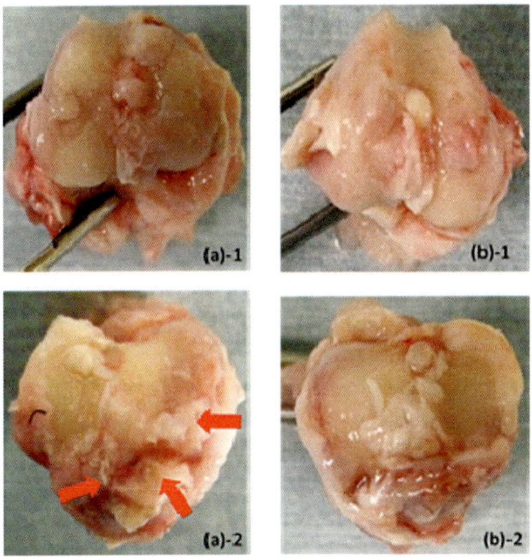

Figure 6.9 Macroscopic appearance of the cartilage surface of knee joints: [(a)-1] Femoral cartilage, [(a)-2] Tibia cartilage in control group, [(b)-1] Femoral cartilage, and [(b)-2] Tibia cartilage in PEG group.

the non-injection, then the rabbits were sacrificed, the cartilage of knee were examined macroscopically and histologically.

Figure 6.9 shows each macro-appearance of the articular cartilage in the knee of the control group and PEG injected group (PEG group).

In PEG group, there were no significant changes in the cartilage in both femur and tibia as compared with the cartilage before injection. In contrast, the apparent erosion, some progression of deformation including the cartilage defect (arrows) was observed in tibial cartilage of the control group as shown in Fig. 6.9(a)-2.

Table 6.1 shows the score for evaluation of cartilage using Chang et al. [22]. This score indicates the degree of cartilage damage, the state of normal cartilage result in higher score, which suggests PEG can lubricant prevent the progress of OA.

Figure 6.10 shows the results of the histological photographs of tibial articular cartilage. Although the partial mild disturbance is observed on the cartilage surface in the PEG group, the cartilage

Table 6.1 The score for evaluation of cartilage. Sample number 3

	Femoral condyle cartilage score (/10)			Tibia cartilage score (/10)		
Sample	1	2	3	1	2	3
Control group	4	2	4	10	6	8
PEG group	2	2		4	2	2

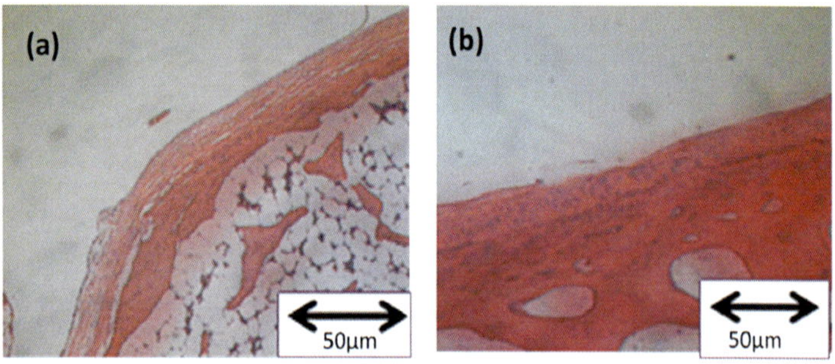

Figure 6.10 Histological appearance of tibia cartilage surfaces (×250): (a) Control group (b) PEG group.

surface itself is maintained. In contrast, control group expose the severe state of cartilage such as thinning and partial delamination.

According to the pathophysiology of OA of knee joint, OA is characterised by a slow degradation of cartilage over several years. In normal cartilage, a delicate balance exists between matrix synthesis and degradation; however, OA cartilage degradation exceeds synthesis or regeneration. The balance is affected and regulated by several factor such as age, weight, etc. Considering that the biomechanical stress also belong to these factor, it would be highly effective for the medication and prevention of OA improving the biomechanical and tribological circumstances for cartilage in knee joint by appropriate lubricant. This experimental result supports this concept.

Moreover, as another mechanism, the interaction between the PEG molecules and the protein in synovial fluid is also suspected. It is well known that the protein, especially albumin in synovial fluid has very important role in boundary lubrication mode in synovial joint. The protein molecules can adsorb on cartilage surface as a wear protective layer, and operate the excellent lubrication system. On the other hand, since PEG molecules are also organic compounds having hydroxyl group (–OH) at both or one end of the molecules, boundary lubricating film would be formed between lubricative surfaces. The improved lubrication mode by two different types of functional lubricants might prevent the OA progress although the detail of mechanism is unclear.

6.4.4 *PEG Lubricant for Protection from Wear of UHMWPE in Artificial Knee Joint*

As another effect of PEG lubricant, the reducing wear of the UHMWPE of artificial knee joint would be expected. In order to access this tribological effect of PEG lubricant, the friction and wear test was performed. This section mainly introduces our works [23, 24].

Using the Co–Cr alloy and UHMWPE sample that were component of current knee prosthesis, the pin-on-disk arranged rotational frictional test was performed as shown in Fig. 6.11. The determined loading condition and frictional mode of this test were much more severe than that of the actual knee prosthesis in vivo.

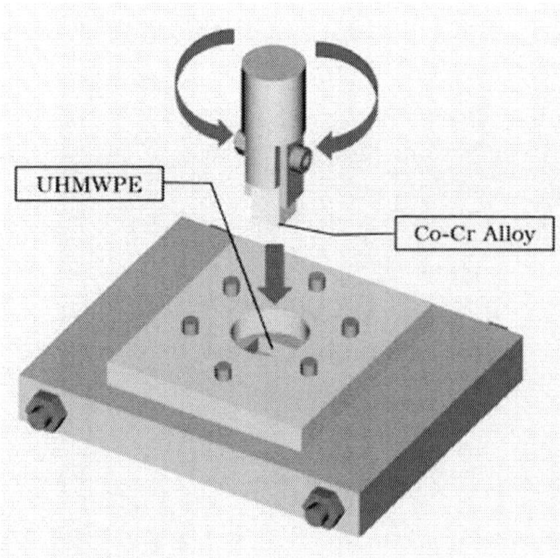

Figure 6.11 The schema of testing device in the rotational frictional test.

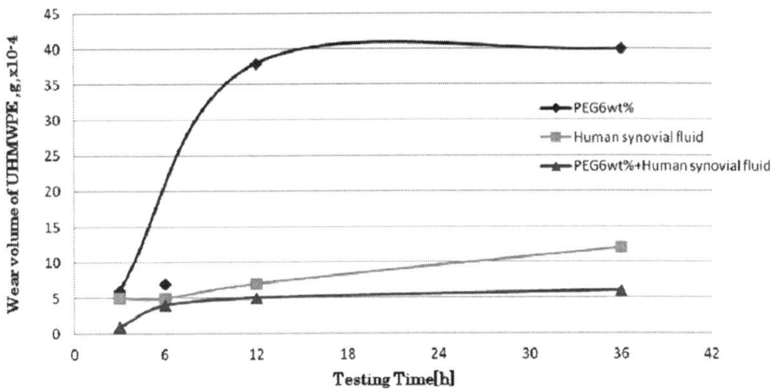

Figure 6.12 The time dependence of the wear volume of UHMWPE in each lubricant in friction test.

For experimental lubricants, the previous PEG lubricant (PEG 6 wt.% hydrate solution), synovial fluid, which is for comparison, and the 50% PEG mixed with 50% human synovial fluid, which is assumed to real clinical articular condition, were selected.

6.4.4.1 Comparison of the amount of wear of UHMWPE

Figure 6.12 shows the time dependence of the wear mass in each lubricant. The HUMWPE wear volume in PEG lubricant increased monotonously with the testing times, while the wear in other lubricants were significantly suppressed, especially, that of the PEG bends with synovial fluid was remarkable.

Figure 6.13 shows the surface of each UHMWPE specimen in the friction testing of 36 hours. The surface in PEG lubricant exposed the considerable damage, many scratched, roughened traces and partial delamination defects were clearly visible. As compared with that, the specimen in PEG mixed synovial fluid lubricant shows good condition including little worn surface with tiny scratch.

6.4.5 *Potential of PEG Lubricant*

Considering that the occurrence of OA is affected by biomechanical stress, the excellent lubrication mode by a sufficient lubricant would be highly effective for the medication and prevention of OA.

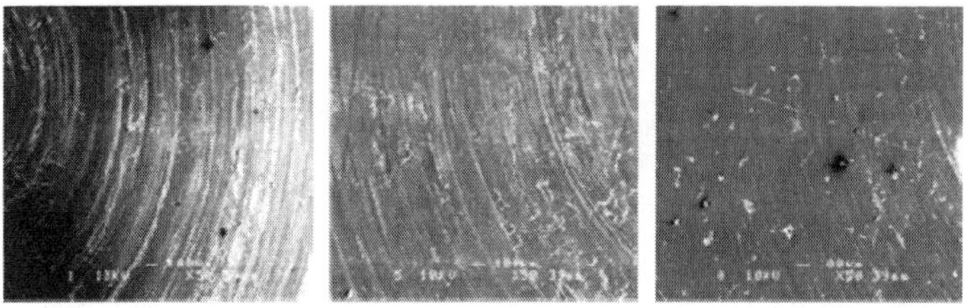

(a) PEG6wt% (b) Human synovial fluid (c) Lubricant mixture

Figure 6.13 The SEM images of surface of UHMWPE in each lubricant in frictional testing (×50)

Highly viscous PEG lubricant was expected to enhance the fluid film lubricating system [25], in even the boundary lubrication, effective boundary lubricating film would be formed between the functional on the metal oxide film of Co–Cr alloy because the hydroxyl group at the ends of the PEG molecules bound more strongly to the metal oxide surface [26].

However, the result of friction test indicated that PEG has no such efficacy under the boundary lubrication in progress in this pin-on-disk arranged test.

On the other hand, the lubricating function of human synovial fluid showed better than that of PEG. Besides, PEG mixed synovial fluid exhibited the most excellent result.

As a lubrication mechanism in this results of frictional test, the formation of the boundary film between the PEG molecules and the protein in synovial fluid is suspected. As mentioned above, the protein molecules in synovial fluid have very important role in boundary lubrication mode in synovial joint. In this protein and PEG molecules complex lubricant, PEG molecules might enhance and strengthen the wear protective layer by proteins between metal and UHMWPE surfaces.

The good result in animal test could not only be due to high viscosity of PEG but also due to interactional mechanism between PEG and protein in synovial fluid.

From the results of our two studies that the blend lubricant of the PEG hydraulic fluid and synovial fluid could be effective for protection of OA progress and wear of UHMWPE, the intra-articular injection method of PEG seems to be promising medical treatment because actual intra-injected PEG inevitably mixed the synovial fluid in knee joint.

Further, study regarding the detail of lubrication mechanism in the synovial fluid and PEG-mixed lubricant should be necessary. In future, by modifying other functional compounds at both or one end of the PEG molecules, more excellent intra-articular injection of PEG lubricant could be developed for OA treatment and longevity of artificial joint of knee.

6.5 Development of PEG as an Artificial Auricular Cartilage

Previous topics mentioned above are concerning the application using PEG sol to current therapy, conservative and surgical treatment for OA of the knee joint. Furthermore, there is more aggressive and advanced study to synthesise a new articular cartilage material using PEG.

As already presented previously, the synovial articular cartilage is composed of proteoglycan attached to a backbone of hyaluronic acid intertwined among the hydrogel network structure of type collagen. This characteristic structure might affect its excellent lubricating function. Although this lubricating mechanism are still unclear, if the artificial cartilage with the excellent lubricating function similar to that of synovial cartilage is developed by using hydrogels, current major issue regarding the durability of artificial knee joint by wear of UHMWPE will be overcome.

Under this concept, many researchers have already tried to develop the ideal artificial articular cartilage using various kinds of polymeric materials, Sakai et al. have successfully designed and fabricated the novel artificial articular cartilage with high mechanical properties using tetra-PEG gel [5, 27]. Generally, hydrogels are defined as 3D polymer networks cross-linked by physical or chemical interaction in water component and show the fragility and low mechanical strength, which come from the micro-inhomogeneity of polymer network structure created by cross-linking. Micro-inhomogeneity is categorised into spatial, topological, connectivity and motility inhomogeneities. As the networks cannot

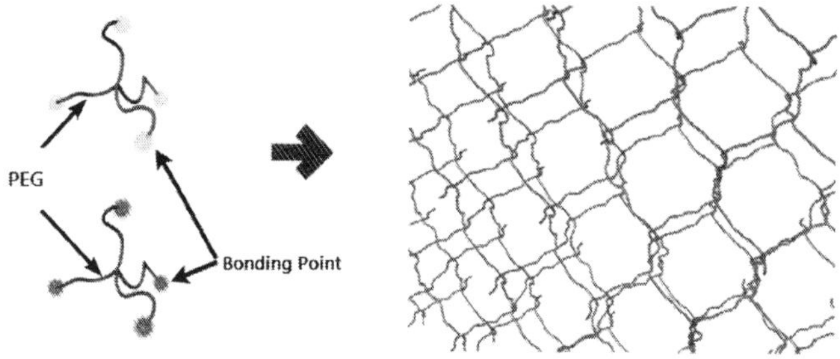

Figure 6.14 The scheme of fabrication process of tetra-PEG network. Reprinted with permission from Ref. [27].

behave cooperatively due to these inhomogeneities, they begin to break from the weakest link, thus reducing the whole mechanical strength.

For this fault of hydrogels, Sakai et al. designed and fabricated a novel homogeneous hydrogel by combing two symmetrical tetrahedron-like PEG macromonomers of the same size. This gel's network, the tetra-network, is made by cross-end-coupling of tetra-PEG arm polymer modules and an extremely homogenous (Fig. 6.14). Because the tetra network can behave as uniformly packed elastic blobs, its cooperativeness equalises the stress distribution; the mechanical strength of this PEG gel is extremely increased, being comparable to that of articular cartilage.

Furthermore, remarkable point is a possibility of fixation to bone tissue. We have also developed an artificial cartilage using polyvinyl alcohol–hydrogel (PVA–H), which has confirmed the mechanical properties, excellent lubricative function. However, this PVA-H has superior bio-inert properties, and hardly adheres or binds to the nature bone, thus firm fixation method of PVA-H is the current problem for the clinical application [28–30].

In contrast, as mentioned before, PEG is able to form the functional bio-interface and excellent biocompatible surface by linking some organic group. Although the details of the durability in vivo and the lubrication function as an articular cartilage of this material are still unknown, PEG gel seems to have a potential to be substitute for cartilage in clinical field.

6.6 Conclusion

The aim of this article is to give an overview over the properties of PEG which are relevant for their applications in orthopaedic surgery and to show the advantages. PEG is very interesting and promising material, by modifying PEG molecules, which have been designed and reconstructed, the hydrated gel structural and functional features such as mechanical strength, tribological character as described above. The appearance of medical application of PEG gels with excellent characteristics in orthopaedic field is expected in future.

Acknowledgements

The author would like to thank Dr. Yoshitaka Nakanishi, Professor of Kumamoto University for giving the opportunity to introduce own study.

References

1. Yamamuro T, Onishi H (1992) *Manual of Orthopaedic Materials*, 1st ed. Kanehara & Co., Ltd., Tokyo, Japan.
2. Hayashi K, Ishii Y, Ninomiya S, Takaoka K, Nakamura T (1997) *Orthopaedic Surgery*, 48(8), Nankoudo Co. Ltd., Tokyo, Japan.
3. Nagasaki Y (2011) Construction of a densely poly(ethylene glycol)-chain-tethered surface and its performance. *Polym J* 43, 949–958.
4. Wittmann C (2006) *Immobilisation of DNA on Chips II (Topics in Current Chemistry)* 1st ed. Springer, NY, USA.
5. Sakai T, Matsunaga T, Yamamoto Y, Ito C, Yoshida R, Suzuki S, Sakai N, Shibayama M, Chung U-I (2008) Design and fabrication of a high-strength hydrogel with ideally homogeneous network structure from tetahedron-like macromonomers. *Macromolecules* 41, 5379–5384.
6. Rahman CV, Kuhn G, White LJ, Kirby GT, Varghese OP, McLaren JS, Cox HC, Rose FR, Müller R, Hilborn J, Shakesheff KM (2013) PLGA/PEG-hydrogel composite scaffolds with controllable mechanical properties. *J Biomed Mater Res B*, DOI: 10.1002/jbm.b.32867

7. Nagasaki Y (2008) PEG-b-polymeric stabilized bionanoparticles for nanodiagnostics and nanotherapy. *Chem Soc Jap* 37, 564–569.
8. Saha N, Saarai A, Roy N, Kitano T, Saha P (2011) Polymeric biomaterial-based hydrogels for biomedical, *Appl J Biomat Nanobiotech* 2, 85–90.
9. Zhang I, Shung KK, Edwards DA (1996) Hydrogels with enhanced mass transfer for transdermal drug delivery. *J Pharm Sci* 85, 1312–1316.
10. Knop K, Hoogenboom R, Fischer D, Schubert US (2010) Poly(ethylene glycol) in drug delivery: Pros and cons as well as potential alternatives. *Angew Chem Int Ed* 49, 6288–6308.
11. Gaoa X, Taoa W, Lua W, Zhanga Q, Zhangb Y, Jianga X, Fu S (2006) Lectin-conjugated PEG–PLA nanoparticles: Preparation and brain delivery after intranasal administration. *Biomaterials* 27, 3482–3490.
12. Yoshiya S (2011) The design and biomechanics of artificial knee joint. *J Joint Surg* 30. Medicalview Co., Tokyo, Japan.
13. Bauer TW, Saitarelli M, Mcmohan JT, Wilde AH (1993) Regional dissemination of wear debris from total knee prosthesis. *J Bone Jt Surg* 75, 106–111.
14. Moskowitz RW, Howell DS, Golgberg VM, Mankin HJ (1992) *Osteoarthritis/Diagnosis and Medical/Surgical Management*, 2nd ed. W. B. Saunders Co., St. Louis, USA.
15. Moreland LW (2003). Intra-articular hyaluronan (hyaluronic acid) and hylans for the treatment of osteoarthritis: Mechanisms of action. *Arthritis Res Ther* 5, 54–67.
16. Goto M, Hanyu T, Yoshino T, Matsuno H, Shimizu M, Murata N, Shiozawa S, Matsubara T, Yamana S, Matsuda T (2001) Intra-articular injection of hyaluronate (SL-6601D) improves joint pain and synovial fluid prostaglandin E2 levels in rheumatoid arthritis: A multicenter clinical trial. *Clin Exper Rheum* 19, 377–383.
17. Neustadt DH (2003) Long-term efficacy and safety of intra-articular sodium hyaluronate (Hyalgen) in patients with osteoarthritis of the knee. *Clin Exper Rheum* 21, 307–311.
18. Tomita N, Kitakura T, Onmori N (1999) Prevention of fatigue cracks in ultrahigh molecular weight polyethylene joint components by the addition of Vitamin E. *J Biomed Res* 48, 474–478.
19. Moro T, Takatori Y, Ishihara K (2004) Surface grafting of artificial joints with a biocompatible polymer for preventing periprostheticosteolysis. *Nature Mater* 3, 829–836.

20. Kobayashi M, Ohashi A, Hyon SY (2013) Assessment of polyethylene glycol as an intra-articular injection for osteoarthritis of knee joint (in Japanese). *Japan J Clinic Biomech* 33, 231–236.
21. Kobayashi M, Kondo M, Hyon SY (2011) Efficacy of tribology function of joint lubricant for the treatment of osteoarthritis knee joint (The evaluation in animal experiment using rabbits) (in Japanese). *Trans Japan Soc Mech Eng* 33, 247–251.
22. Chang YS, Oka M, Gu HO, Kobayashi M, Toguchida J, Nakamura T, Hayami T (1997) Histologic comparison of tibial articular surfaces against rigid materials and artificial articular cartilage. *J Biomed Mater Res* 37, 51–59.
23. Kobayashi M, Honda Y, Hyon SY (2013) Development of artificial Intra-articular lubricant using polyethylene glycol (PEG) (evaluation war of ultra-high molecular weight polyethylene (UHMWPE))(in Japanese). *Japan J Clinic Biomech* 33, 251–256.
24. Honda Y, Kobayashi M, Matsumura K, Nakajima N, Hyon S-H (2011) Development of artificial intra-articular polyethtleneglycol (PEG) lubricant for survival of total knee joint patient; preliminary study for clinical application. *Proceedings of the 11th International IEEE Conference on Bioinformatics and Bioengineering (BIBE), IEEE Comp Soc*, 121–124. DOI: 10.1109/BIBE.2011.26
25. Sakurai T (1991) *Tribology Series 1*, 2nd ed. Saiwai Press, Japan.
26. Okabe H, Masuko M, Sakuai K (1981) Dynamic behavior of surface-adsorbed molecules under boundary lubrications. *Trans ASLE* 24, 467–473.
27. Sakai T, Akagi Y, Matsunaga T, Kurakazu M, Chung U-I, Shibayama M (2010) Highly elastic and deformable hydrogel formed from tetra-arm polymers. *Macromol Rapid Commun* 31, 1954–1959.
28. Noguchi T, Oka M, Yamamuro T (1991) Poly vinyl alcohol hydrogels as an artificial articular cartilage: Evaluation of biocompatibility. *J Appl Biomater* 2, 101–107.
29. Kobayashi M, Oka M (2004) Characterization of a polyvinyl alcohol-hydrogel artificial articular cartilage prepared by injection-molding. *J Biomater Sci Polymer Ed* 15, 741–751.
30. Kobayashi M, Oka M (2004) Composite device for attachment of PVA-H to underlying bone. *Artif Organs* 28, 734–738.

Chapter 7

Environmentally Friendly Bearing and Sealing Systems with Artificial Articular Cartilage for Power Generation from Natural Energy

Yoshitaka Nakanishi

Graduate School of Science and Technology, Kumamoto University, 2-39-1 Kurokami, Kumamoto 860-8555, Japan

y-naka@mech.kumamoto-u.ac.jp

7.1 Introduction

Renewable energy research and its application have been promoted to slow down climate change and maintain economic growth. Streamflow or tidal power is valued as a source of energy, and environmentally friendly and low-friction *bearing* and sealing systems that employ biomimetic technologies are proposed for its utilisation. The proposed system is referred to as 'Bio-Star', an abbreviation for **Bio**mimetic **S**ystem for **T**idal power generation learned from **Ar**ticular cartilage. A dynamo-electric generator and ancillary systems with waterproof construction are installed near or under

Hydrated Materials: Applications in Biomedicine and the Environment
Edited by Yoshitaka Nakanishi

ISBN 978-981-4463-22-5 (Hardcover), 978-981-4463-23-2 (eBook)
www.panstanford.com

water. Lip seals with rotating shaft prevent the ingress of water from the outside, and excellent frictional properties with various rotation speeds are required to improve the power generation efficiency with constantly changing water flow. The Bio-Star was successfully developed using a hydrated material (polyvinyl formal; PVF) that mimics articular cartilage in a natural synovial joint. Polyethylene glycol (PEG) dissolved in distilled water, which is a non-Newtonian fluid, was used as a lubricant. These materials have low toxicity and low environmental impact. The biomimetic sealing system exhibits excellent frictional properties with extremely low ingress of water.

7.2 Clustered Micro-Generation System for Streamflow and Tidal Power Generation

A clustered micro-generation system has been developed for performance assessment of the Bio-Star (Fig. 7.1). Each individual

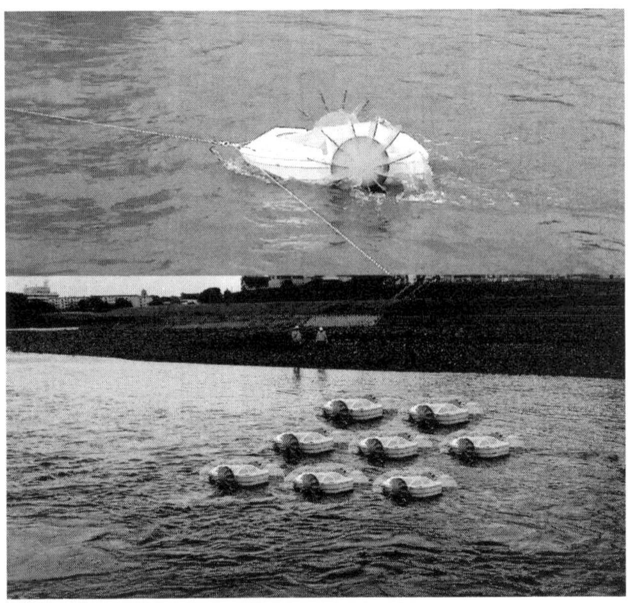

Figure 7.1 Demonstration of streamflow generation and image of clustered micro-generation system.

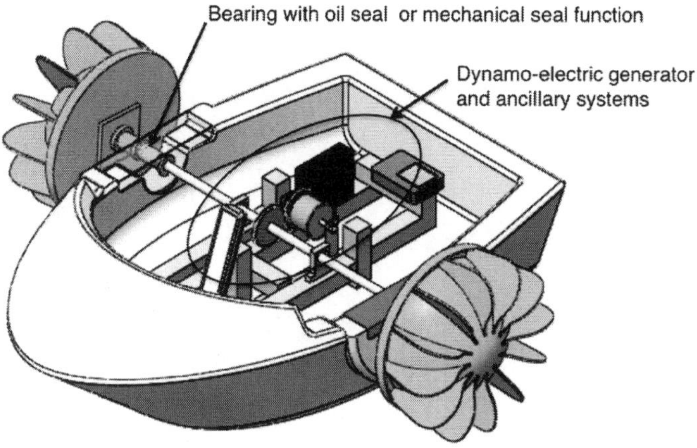

Figure 7.2 Schematic illustration of micro-generation.

generation unit is small and light (length: 1.2 m, width: 1.0 m, height: 0.8 m, weight: 20 kg) and can be easily placed or removed without the need for related infrastructure construction. A large amount of power can be generated by combining a number of generation units, and the total power generation is not significantly affected if one unit breaks down or is deactivated for maintenance. The dynamo-electric generator and ancillary systems are installed inside the floating body and have a waterproof construction (Fig. 7.2). The Bio-Star (Type 1: bearing system), which supports a rotating shaft, should function to prevent the ingress of water from the outside, in addition to having excellent frictional properties to improve the power generation efficiency under constantly changing water flow. A next-generation micro-generation system that will generate more electrical energy is currently under development (Fig. 7.3). This system has two rotating shafts in contact with the water flow, so that a new sealing system (Bio-Star, Type 2: sealing system) with extremely low ingress of water and low friction is required.

7.3 'Bio-Star': Bearing and Seal System

To achieve the specification requirements for the micro-generation system, a sealing and lubrication system that mimics a natural

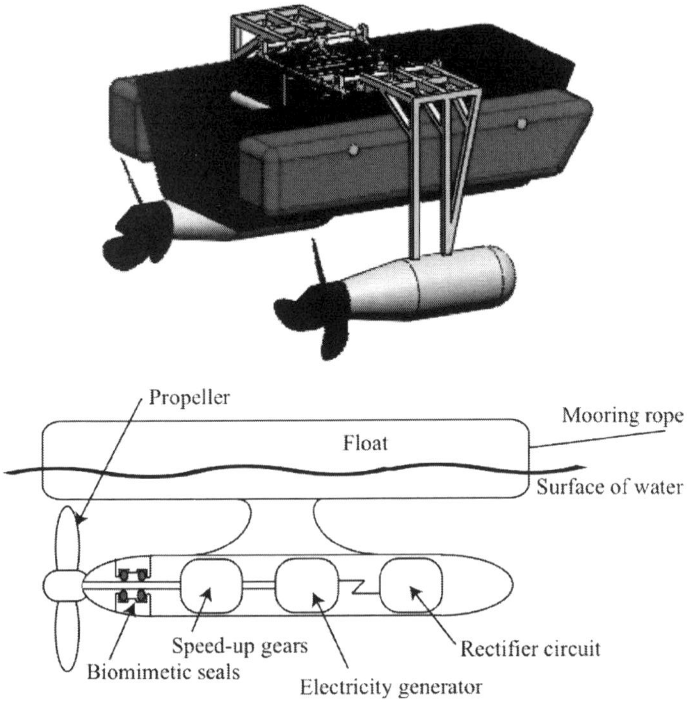

Figure 7.3 Schematic illustration of next- generation streamflow generation unit. All-new sealing system with extremely low leakage of water and friction is installed in the generation unit.

synovial joint was developed. It is considered that the widely varying loads and sliding speeds found in synovial joints are accommodated by a combination of lubrication mechanisms that involve both synovial fluid and articular cartilage (Fig. 7.4) [1]. Such lubrication has been modelled in terms of hydrodynamic lubrication [2]; the softness of cartilage, in comparison to that of typical engineering materials, may facilitate elastohydrodynamic lubrication. A weeping lubrication model was also proposed, in which synovial fluid is temporarily stored inside the cartilage and released during periods of high contact load. The ability of synovial fluid to depart from Newtonian rheology, in which the viscosity increases with decreasing shear rate, may prevent contact between opposing cartilage surfaces in the boundary lubrication mode.

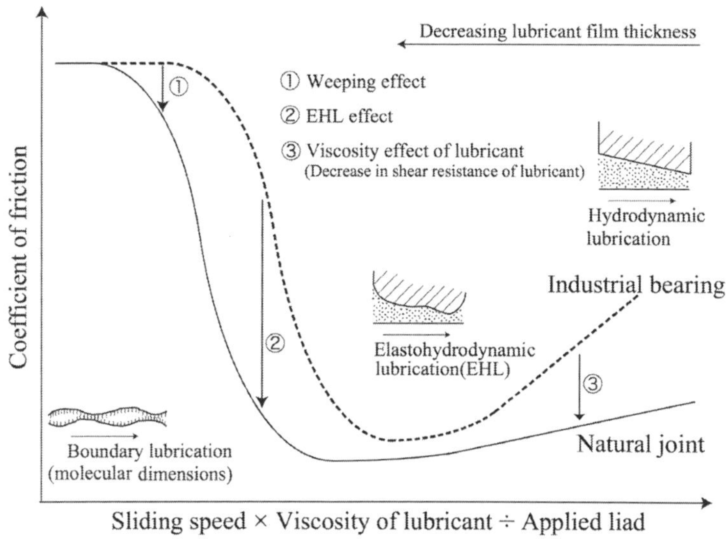

Figure 7.4 Frictional characteristics of an industrial seal and a natural synovial joint.

Furthermore, non-Newtonian behaviour has the potential to reduce the friction in the full fluid film lubrication mode because the shear resistance of the fluid is reduced in accordance with the increase in its shear rate.

Attempts have been made to investigate and artificially reproduce the system of lubrication in natural synovial joints. Typical application areas are in the medical field [3–5], in which next-generation joint prostheses are expected to demonstrate ultralow friction and wear. The proposed environmentally friendly sealing system produces low friction in various lubrication modes and has the potential for application in systems such as a streamflow or tidal power generation systems (Fig. 7.3), where mechanical loss should be reduced to increase power generation efficiency and marine pollution should be avoided.

The hydration lubrication that is observed in articular cartilage has been frequently reproduced using gels or porous materials as bearing materials. One such material is a polyvinyl alcohol (PVA) hydrogel, which is one of the few polymers with hydrophilic

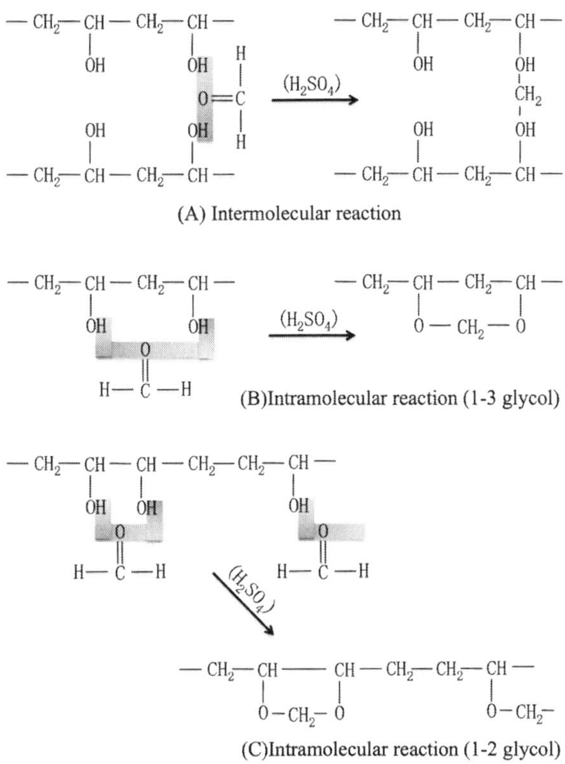

Figure 7.5 Chemical reactions for the formation of PVF from PVA. Adapted from Nakanishi et al. [6].

properties. However, PVA hydrogel has a shortcoming in that it has low wear resistance. Therefore, improvement of the wear resistance was attempted by performing a chemical cross-linking reaction of PVA to produce PVF as a bearing or sealing material for the Bio-Star system [6].

Figure 7.5 shows the chemical reaction for the formation of PVF from PVA. When PVA is reacted with formaldehyde (HCHO) together with an acid catalyst (H_2SO_4), it is converted into PVF, which exhibits water-resistant properties and excellent mechanical properties. During the formalisation reaction, intermolecular formaldehydes react with PVA molecules and simultaneous intramolecular reactions occur, where formaldehyde reacts with 1-2

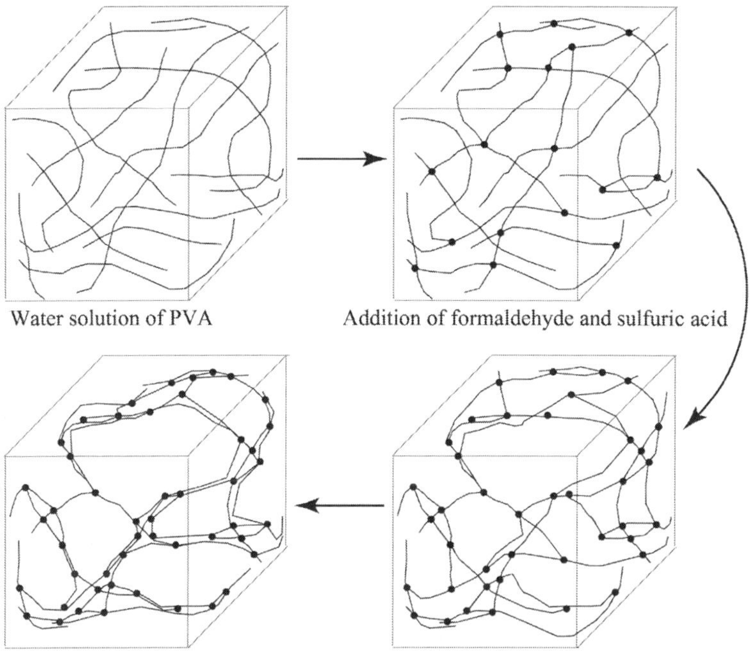

Figure 7.6 Formation of PVF as a continuous porous body. Adapted from Nakanishi et al. [6].

glycols and 1-3 glycols within one molecule. The resulting PVF is a co-polymer that consists of a mixture of alcoholic hydroxyl groups, acetyl groups, and formal groups.

Figure 7.6 shows the process for PVF formation on a microscopic scale. PVA dissolved in water is subjected to intermolecular formalisation, which results in an enhancement of cross-linking between principal chains of the polymer. Formalisation also proceeds intra-molecularly, so that the principal chains of the polymer prevent transformation into insoluble PVF. However, hydrophilicity is preserved, due to the presence of residual alcoholic hydroxyl groups that do not participate in the reaction. Water is removed during the reaction process and the principal polymer chains aggregate by intermolecular forces, which results in the formation of pores and a 3D network of beams. The PVF formed by this process

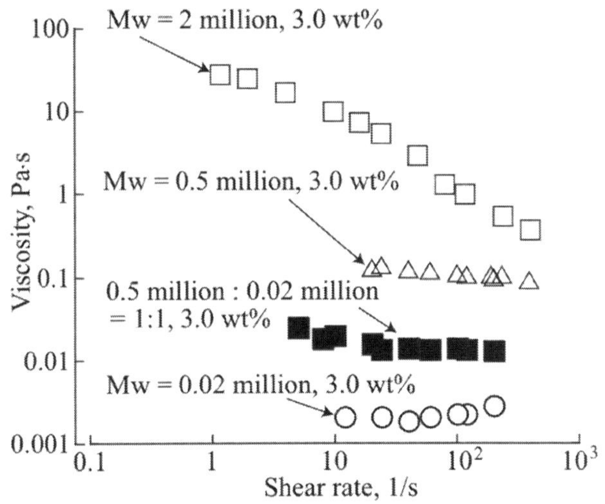

Figure 7.7 Viscosities of PEG lubricants.

is hydrophilic and has a continuously porous structure, which is considered to significantly promote hydration lubrication.

An aqueous solution of PEG was used as a lubricant for the Bio-Star system. PEG with molecular weights of 0.02 million, 0.5 million, and 2.0 million was employed. The PEG was hydrated by dissolving in distilled water at 48°C with stirring for 48 hours. Figure 7.7 shows the viscosities of the PEG lubricants measured using a cone–plate viscometer. The higher molecular weight PEG exhibited more non-Newtonian characteristics, in which the viscosity decreased with increase in the shear rate. The viscosity of a mixed PEG lubricant was intermediate between the two individual molecular weight lubricants.

Figure 7.8 shows the testing apparatus for the Bio-Star (Type 2 sealing system). A 30 mm diameter stainless steel (SUS304, JIS) shaft with a surface finish of 0.02 μm (Ra) is used. Two lip seals (40 mm OD, 30 mm ID, 5 mm thick) are moulded from PVF with a pore diameter of 5 μm and are lubricated with PEG lubricant to separate the water and gas phases. Oil seals (AE1709A, Nok Corp., Japan) and a mechanical sealing system (CCU30-PAP00-303, Nippon Pillar Co., Ltd., Japan) in popular use are also compared with the

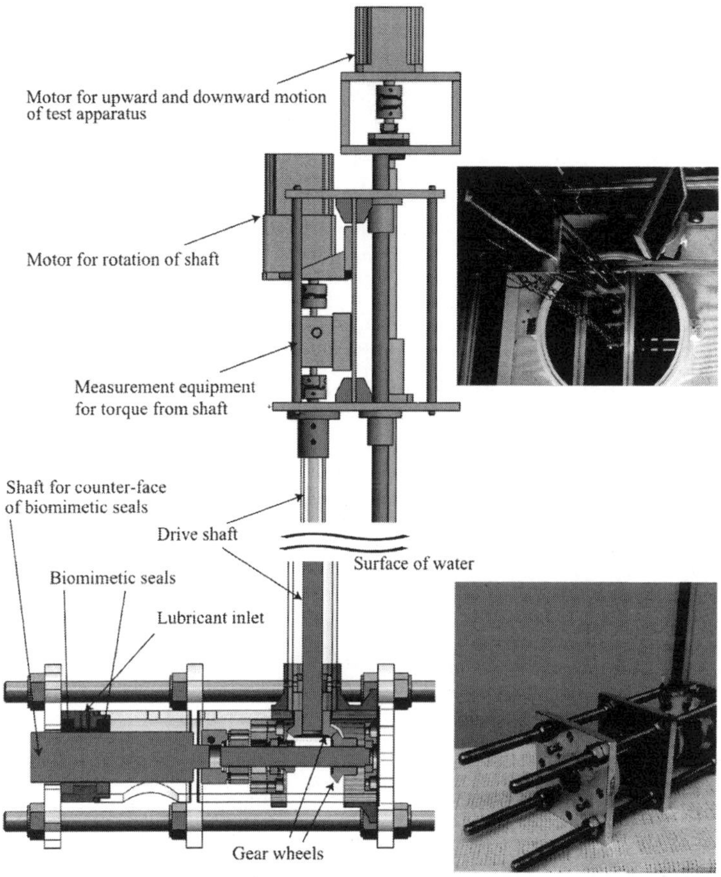

Figure 7.8 Testing apparatus for the Bio-Star (Type 2 sealing system).

PVF lip seals. The shaft rotates at 20 rpm at a water depth of 0.75 m and the direction of shaft rotation was changed every hour. The frictional torque and ingress rate from the water phase were measured. The water ingress rate is calculated as the difference between the amount of liquid that flows into the testing apparatus and the amount of lubricating liquid used for lubrication.

The frictional torque and ingress rate for each sealing system are shown in Fig. 7.9. The biomimetic lip seals (Bio-Star, Type 2) have extremely low ingress of water with lower friction than the

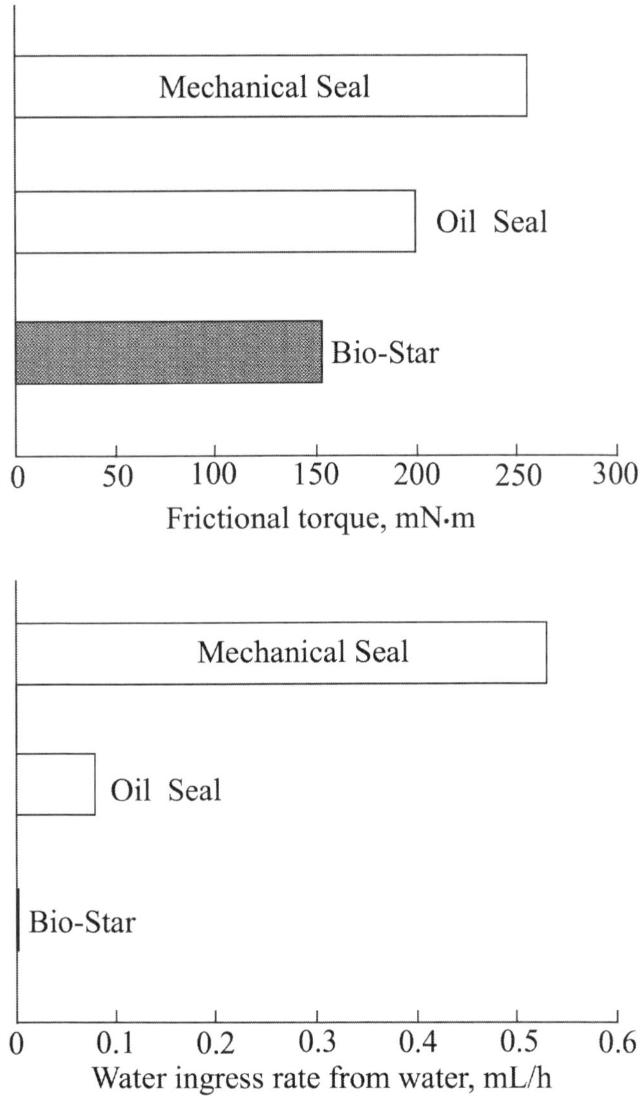

Figure 7.9 Frictional torque and water ingress rate in each sealing system. PEG lubricant (Mw = 2 million, 3 wt%) was used in Bio-Star (Type 2 sealing system).

oil and mechanical seals examined. This result suggests that the biomimetic sealing system is promising for streamflow or tidal power generation applications.

Acknowledgements

This project was supported by the New Energy and Industrial Technology Development Organisation (NEDO) of Japan.

References

1. Batchelor AW, Stachowiak GW (1991) Arthritis and the interacting mechanisms of synovial joint lubrication. Part 2: Joint lubrication and its relation to arthritis, *Orthop Rheumatol*, 9, 11–21.
2. Ochsner A, Waquar A (2010) Biomechanical testing of orthopedic implants: aspects of tribology and simulation, in *Biomechanics of Hard Tissues* (Nakanishi Y, ed), Willey-VCH Verlag GmbH & Co. KGaA, Weinheim, 145–157.
3. Dowson D, Fisher J, Jin ZM, Auger DD, Jobbins B (1991) Design considerations of cushion form bearing in artificial hip joints, *Proc Instn Mech Engrs H*, 205, 59–68.
4. Auger DD, Dowson D, Fisher J (1995) Cushion form bearings for total knee joint replacement, Part 1: Design, friction and lubrication, *Proc Instn Mech Engrs H*, 209, 73–81.
5. Oka M, Ushio K, Kumar P, Ikeuchi K, Hyon SH, Nakamura T, Fujita H (2000) Development of artificial articular cartilage, *Proc Instn Mech Engrs H*, 214, 59–68.
6. Nakanishi Y, Takashima T, Higaki H, Shimoto K, Umeno T, Miura H, Iwamoto Y (2009) Development of biomimetic bearing with hydrated materials, *J Biomech Sci Eng*, 4(2), 249–264.

Chapter 8

Controlling Water-Based or Oil-Based Film between Shoes and the Floor to Prevent Slips and Falls

Takeshi Yamaguchi and Kazuo Hokkirigawa
Graduate School of Engineering, Tohoku University, 6-01, 6-chome, Aramaki-Aza-Aoba, Aoba-ku Sendai-shi, Miyagi 980-8579, Japan
yamatake@gdl.mech.tohoku.ac.jp

8.1 Introduction

Falls are the leading cause of occupational accidents in Japan [1]. Slips are the most frequent event leading to falling accidents [2–5]. Most accidents that involve slips and falls in a work place occur on liquid-contaminated floor surfaces [6–8]. Floor surfaces are often contaminated with water or oil in food factories and restaurant kitchens, causing slips because of the formation of a fluid film on the contact interface between the soles of shoes and the floor surface. Therefore, a footwear outsole pattern is required that is very resistant to slipping on floor surfaces covered with water or oil.

A high static coefficient of friction (SCOF) and a dynamic coefficient of friction (DCOF) are needed at the shoe–floor interface

Hydrated Materials: Applications in Biomedicine and the Environment
Edited by Yoshitaka Nakanishi

ISBN 978-981-4463-22-5 (Hardcover), 978-981-4463-23-2 (eBook)
www.panstanford.com

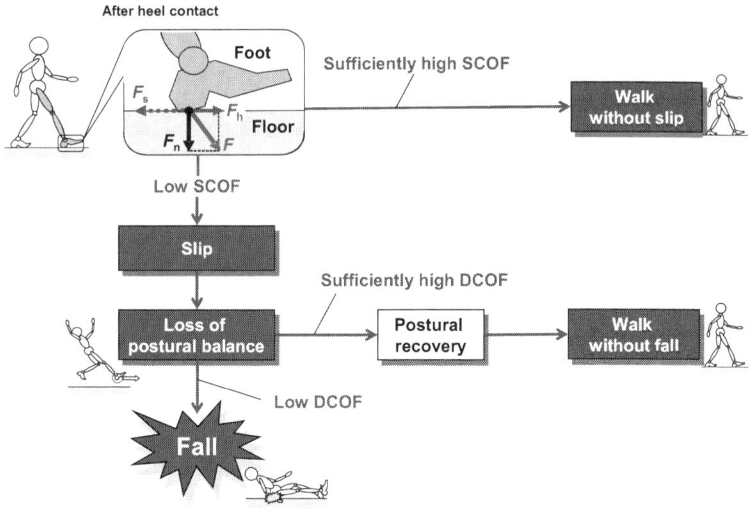

Figure 8.1 Schematic diagram of the relationship between slip-related falls and the coefficient of friction at the shoe–floor interface.

during walking to prevent slip initiation and to stop a slip if it occurs (Fig. 8.1). Previous biomechanical studies on the safety limits of SCOF and DCOF [9–14] indicated that SCOF and DCOF values greater than 0.4 are required at the shoe–floor interface to prevent a slip (and hence a fall) during level walking.

Surface pattern designs of footwear outsoles, including the tread pattern (macroscopic pattern) and surface roughness (microscopic pattern), are helpful to drain liquid from the shoe–floor interface to increase slip resistance, that is, the coefficient of friction [6, 15–19]. However, the design criteria for a shoe sole pattern with sufficiently high SCOF and DCOF on contaminated surfaces are unclear. A new rubber surface pattern was developed by Yamaguchi et al. [20] to increase both the SCOF and DCOF by removing fluid film from the contact interface.

This section describes the main research results of the rubber surface pattern that was designed to remove fluid film from the contact interface and the development of a strong grip shoe outsole that uses the surface pattern [21].

8.2 Hybrid Rubber Surface Pattern to Increase SCOF and DCOF when Lubricated by a Water-Based Lubricant

Yamaguchi et al. [20] found that a rectangular rubber block with a smooth surface (Ra = 0.98 μm) has low SCOF and high steady-state DCOF values, as shown in Fig. 8.2(a), whereas a rubber block with a rough surface (Ra = 30.4 μm) has high SCOF and low steady-state DCOF values on a smooth stainless steel surface (Ra = 0.09 μm) covered with 90% water solution of glycerol (viscosity, η: 224 mPas), as shown in Fig. 8.2(b).

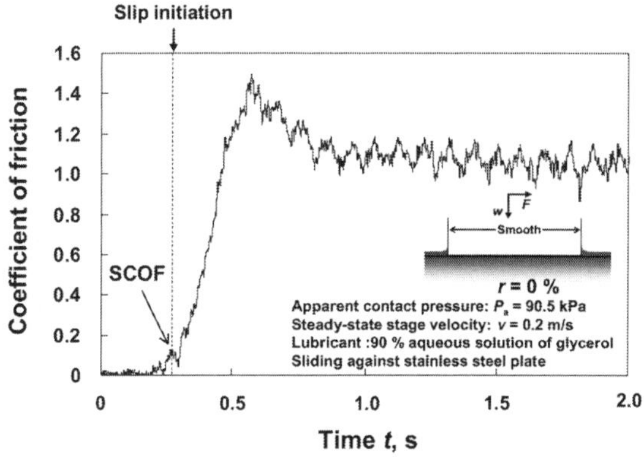

(a) A rectangular rubber block with a smooth surface (Ra = 0.98 μm)

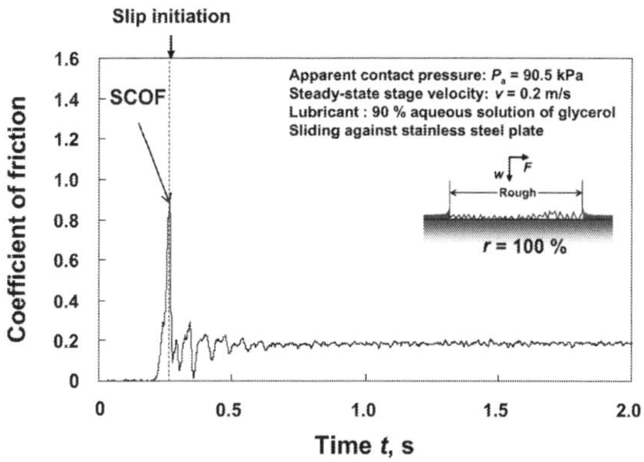

(b) A rectangular rubber block with a rough surface (Ra = 30.4 μm)

Figure 8.2 Variation over time of the coefficient of friction [20].

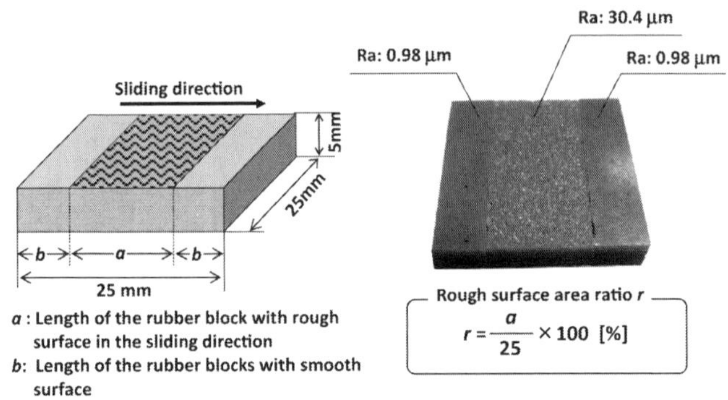

Figure 8.3 Hybrid rubber surface pattern [20].

Based on these findings, they developed a rubber block with a surface pattern of rough and smooth surfaces (a hybrid rubber surface pattern) as shown in Fig. 8.3. The hybrid rubber surface pattern with a rough surface area ratio r of 50% (a ratio of the surface area of the rough surface component to that of a single tread block) provided almost the same values of the SCOF and steady-state DCOF at around 0.5 when lubricated with a glycerol solution lubricant, as shown in Fig. 8.4.

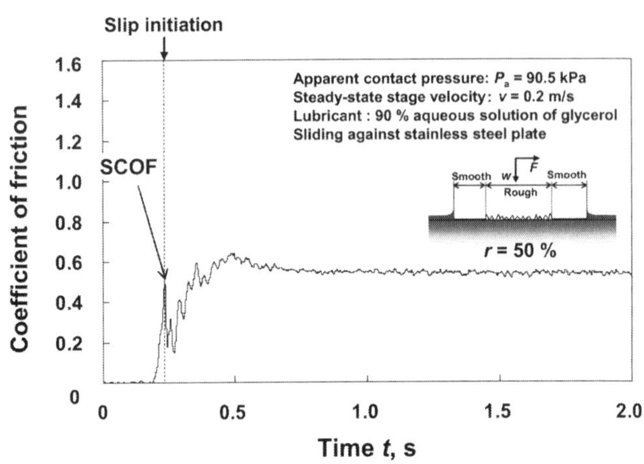

Figure 8.4 Variation over time of the coefficient of friction for the hybrid rubber block with $r = 50\%$ [20].

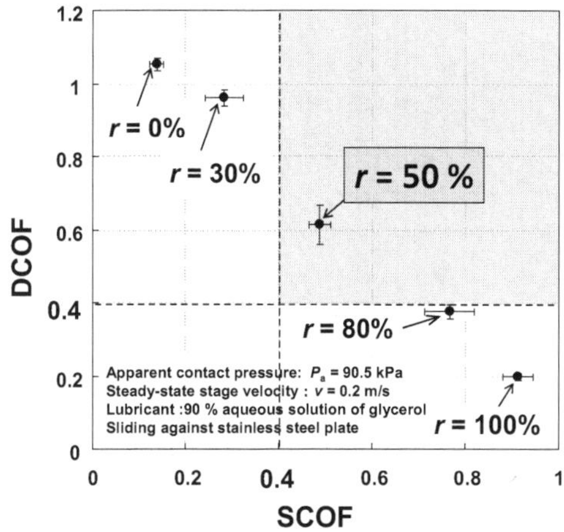

Figure 8.5 Relationship between the static coefficient of friction and the steady-state dynamic coefficient of friction for each rubber block [20].

Figure 8.5 shows the relationship between the values of the SCOF and the steady-state DCOF for a rubber surface pattern with a different rough surface area ratio. The rough surface area ratio $r = 50\%$ achieves SCOF and DCOF values that are greater than 0.4 on a liquid-contaminated surface.

Therefore, the frictional properties obtained by the hybrid rubber block with a rough surface area ratio $r = 50\%$ will be effective in preventing slip occurrence and falling due to an induced slip. The hybrid rubber surface pattern will be applicable to a highly slip-resistant sole pattern for footwear on contaminated surfaces.

8.3 High-Friction Mechanism of a Hybrid Rubber Surface Pattern

To investigate the mechanism of how the hybrid rubber surface pattern achieves increased levels of SCOF and DCOF for a smooth surface covered with a water solution of glycerol, rubber blocks with the hybrid rubber surface pattern were slid against a glass plate with surface roughness Ra of 0.004 μm, which was lubricated with a glycerol solution, and the contact area between the rubber block and

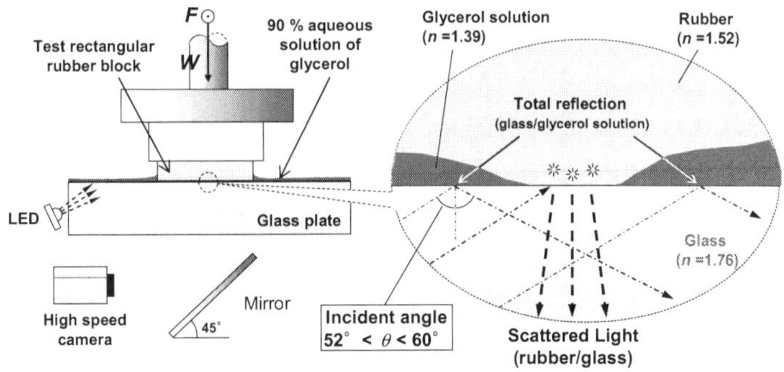

Figure 8.6 Schematic diagram of the measurement principle of the contact area between rubber and glass using the total reflection of light between the glass plate and the glycerol solution; *n* indicates the refractive index.

glass plate surface was measured using the total reflection of light at the contact interface [22].

The total reflection can only occur at the contact interface between the glycerol solution and the glass plate when the angle of incidence is set between 52° and 60° (Fig. 8.6). At these angles of incidence, the contact interface between the rubber block and the glass plate can be observed as a bright section, while the area where the glycerol solution that exists between the rubber and glass appears as a dark section due to the total reflection between the glass and the glycerol solution. Grey-level photographs taken by a high-speed camera were converted to black-and-white binary images.

Figure 8.7(a) represents coefficient of friction as a function of time for the rubber block with a completely smooth surface (r = 0%) and shows the sequential snapshots of the binary images of the contact interface between the rubber block and the glass plate. When the slip initiated, the contact area between the rubber block and the glass plate (white area) was negligible and the SCOF value was very small, because the glycerol solution film existed in the contact interface. Then, the coefficient of friction increased as the contact area increased. Eventually, when sliding was at a steady state, the anterior half part of the rubber block directly contacted with the glass plate and the steady-state DCOF reached a high value around 1.0.

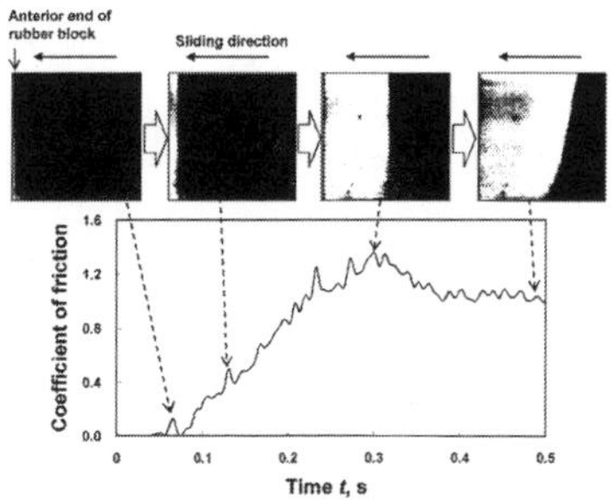

(a) $r = 0\%$

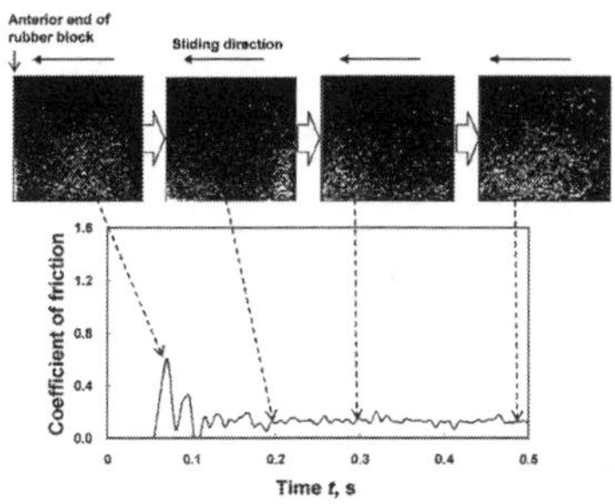

(b) $r = 100\%$

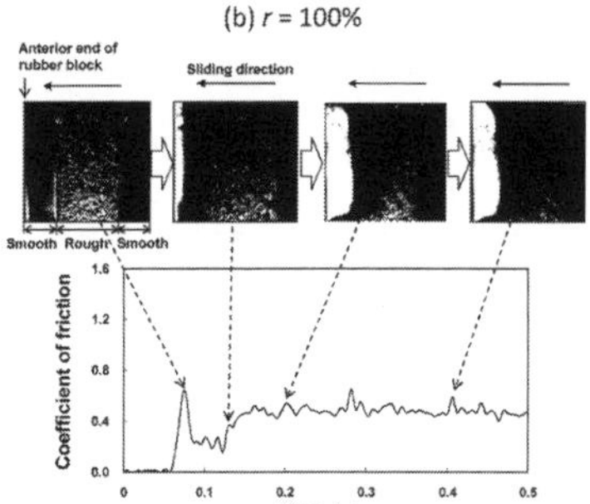

(c) $r = 50\%$

Figure 8.7 Coefficient of friction as a function of time and sequential snapshots of the black-and-white binary images of the contact interface between the rubber and the glass plate; the white sections in the binary images correspond to the contact area between the rubber and glass plate.

On the contrary, for the rubber block with a completely rough surface ($r = 100\%$), the asperities of the rough rubber surface directly contacted with the glass plate both when the slip initiated and during the steady-state sliding, as shown in Fig. 8.7(b). The

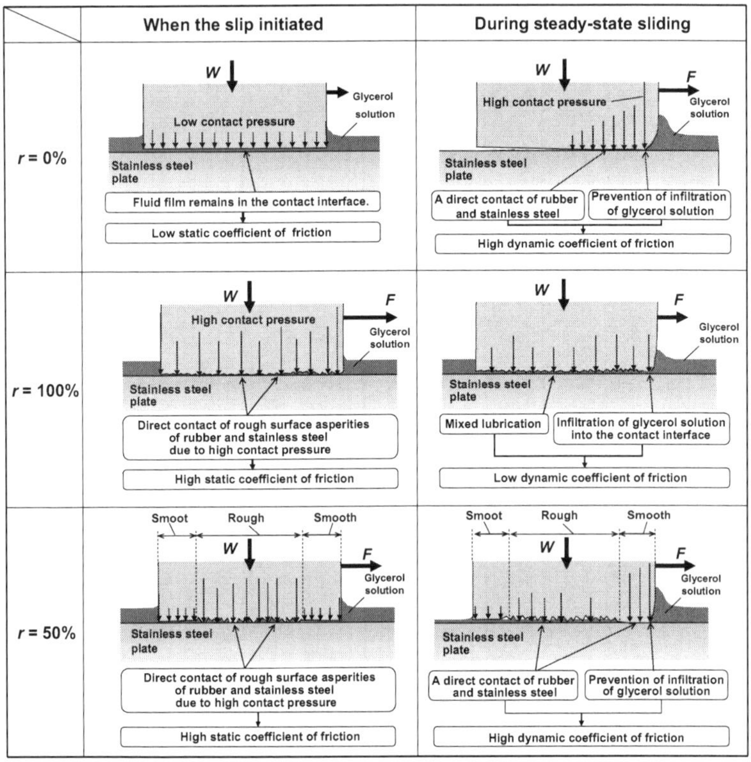

Figure 8.8 Schematic diagram of the contact interface between the rubber blocks with r of 0%, 50%, and 100% and the stainless steel plate contaminated with the glycerol solution [20].

contact area when the slip initiated is clearly greater than that of the rubber block with a completely smooth surface. However, the contact area during the steady-state sliding was smaller than that of the rubber block with a completely smooth surface.

As shown in Fig. 8.7(c), for the hybrid rubber block, only the asperities of the rough rubber surface made direct contact with the glass plate when the slip initiated, which resulted in high SCOF values. The anterior of the smooth rubber surface made direct contact with the glass plate in addition to the asperities of the rough rubber surface during steady-state sliding.

The superior slip resistance of the hybrid rubber surface pattern was achieved by allowing sufficient contact area between the rubber block and the surface, resulting in a removal of glycerol solution film from the contact interface, both when the slip initiated and during the sliding. The results are summarised in Fig. 8.8.

8.4 Development of a Footwear Outsole with a Strong Grip Using a Hybrid Rubber Surface Pattern

On the basis of the results obtained in the fundamental friction tests, footwear was developed with an outsole using a hybrid rubber surface pattern, as shown in Fig. 8.9, and tested to determine its efficacy in increasing slip resistance and reducing the risk of falling due to a slip while walking on a contaminated floor surface.

Figure 8.10 shows the test footwear. Footwear A was a commercially available boot that is conventionally used in food factories and restaurant kitchens (Fig. 8.10a). The comparative footwear had tread blocks with a pear skin-finish surface and a round chamfered edge. Footwear B was a sneaker-type footwear with an outsole of tread blocks and a hybrid rubber surface pattern (Fig. 8.10b). The ratio of the surface area of the rough surface to that of a single tread block (the rough surface area ratio) was 50% for the outsole with the hybrid rubber surface pattern. The outsoles of both types of footwear were made from nitrile butadiene rubber (shore hardness: 58 (A/15) for footwear A; 45 (A/15) for footwear B).

The gait trials on a stainless steel floor covered with a glycerol solution (glycerine concentration: 70 wt.%; viscosity: 19.7 mPas) was carried out with 14 healthy adult males. Figure 8.11 shows the experimental set-up. Subjects were asked to walk straight and turn 180° at the end of the stainless steel floor.

The mean frequency of trials in which a slip occurred is presented in Fig. 8.12 for each type of footwear. The mean frequency of trials with a slip using footwear A and footwear B was 97.6% (41/42) and 66.7% (28/42), respectively. A paired *t*-test indicated that these frequency values were significantly different ($p < 0.05$). Therefore, footwear B reduced the frequency of slip occurrence by 30.9 points compared with footwear A. Such a lower frequency of

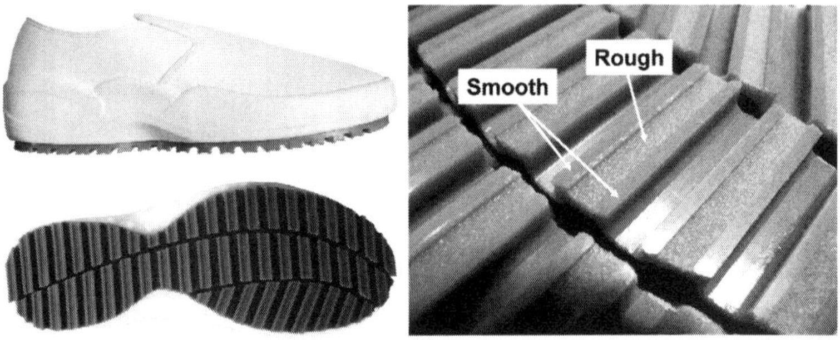

Figure 8.9 The shoe sole pattern by use of the hybrid rubber block (r = 50%).

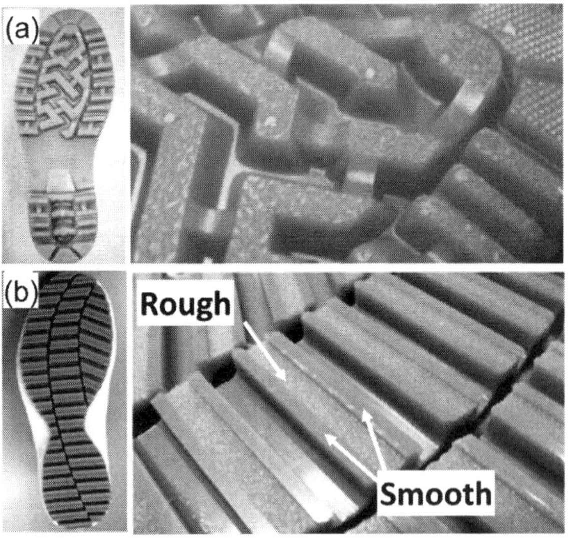

Figure 8.10 Test footwear; (a) footwear A (outsole with tread blocks and a pear skin-finish surface); (b) footwear B (outsole with tread blocks and a hybrid rubber surface pattern).

slip occurrence with footwear B was possibly achieved due to higher SCOF at the shoe–floor interface.

Figure 8.13 shows the relationship between the mean maximum slip distance ($D_{\max}$) and the slip velocity ($v_{\max}$) for both types of footwear. Error bars indicate standard deviations. The paired

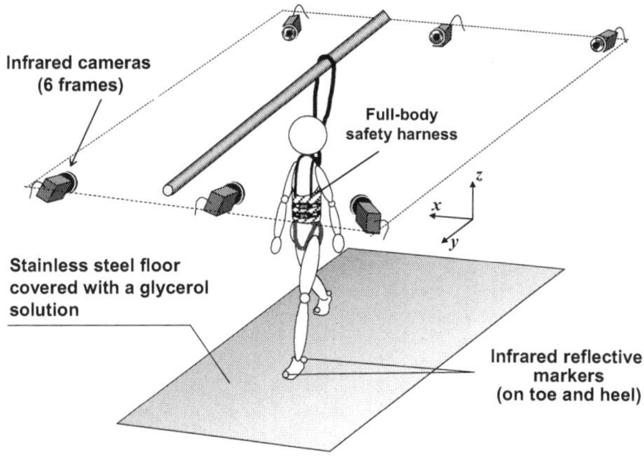

Figure 8.11 Schematic representation of the experimental setup.

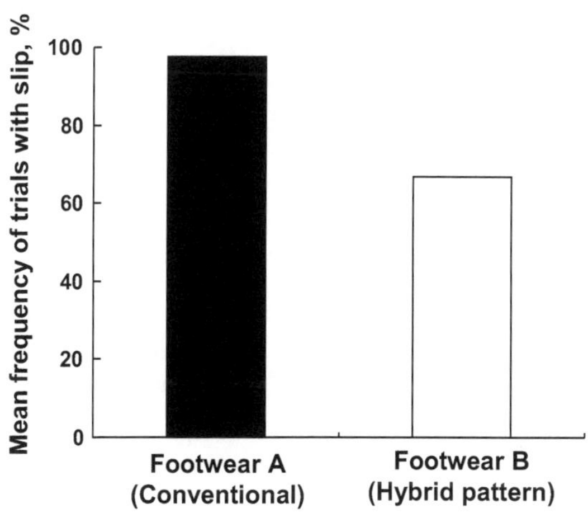

Figure 8.12 Mean frequency of fall trials for both types of footwear.

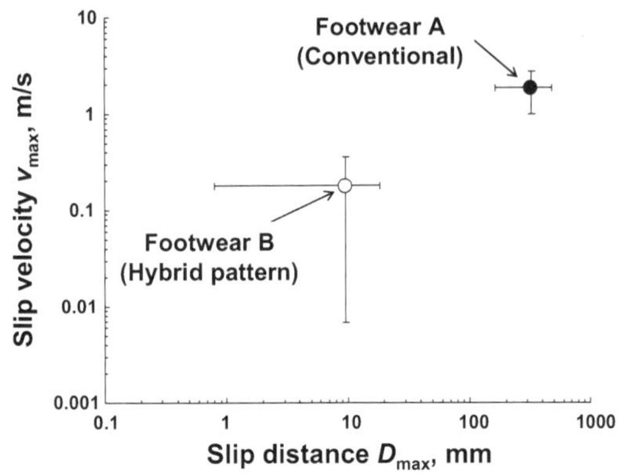

Figure 8.13 Maximum slip distance and maximum slip velocity of the slipping foot for both types of footwear.

t-test indicated that the mean D_{max} and v_{max} values for footwear B were significantly lower than those for footwear A ($p < 0.05$). Footwear B reduced the mean D_{max} and v_{max} values by 97% and 90%, respectively, compared with footwear A ($p < 0.05$). Particularly, the mean slip distance for footwear B was 9.6 mm, which was almost the same as the mean value of the marker fluctuation (6.0 mm); therefore, the slip distance for footwear B was negligibly small. Slip distance and slip velocity are indicators of the risk of falling caused by an induced slip while walking; a greater slip distance and slip velocity are associated with a greater frequency of falls [23–25]. Therefore, a shorter slip distance and a slower slip velocity do not lead to a fall with footwear B. These results could be achieved by a higher DCOF at the shoe–floor interface.

The mean frequency of trials in which a fall occurred for both types of footwear is presented in Fig. 8.14. The frequency of falling during the trials for footwear A and B were 54.8% (23/42) and 0%, respectively; in other words, no subjects fell while testing footwear B.

The measurements of the frequency of slips, slip distance, and slip velocity for the new footwear sole were significantly lower than those for the comparative footwear, which resulted in no falls during the trials.

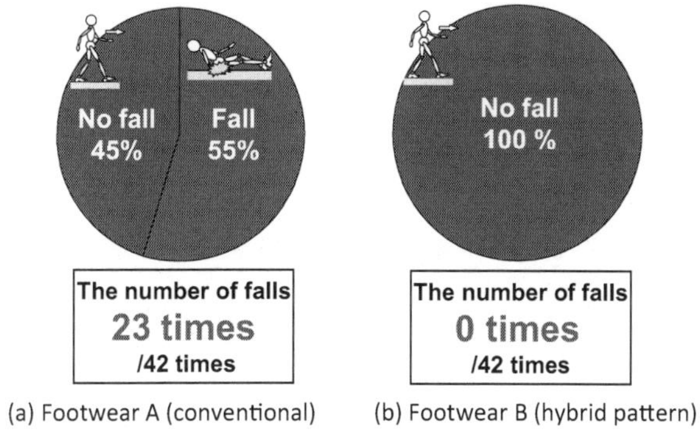

Figure 8.14 Frequency of trials in which a fall occurred.

Superior slip-resistance as well as efficacy in reducing the risk of falling with footwear B, which had the hybrid rubber surface pattern on the tread block of the outsole, was possibly because of the high SCOF and DCOF values of the hybrid rubber surface pattern [20].

As shown in Fig. 8.15(a), when the tread block with the hybrid rubber surface pattern came in contact with a floor covered with a glycerol solution, the glycerol solution film is removed at the contact points due to the high contact pressure of the rough surface asperities, resulting in a direct contact between the asperities of the rough surface component and the stainless steel floor surface. Therefore, the SCOF reached a high value, resulting in a low frequency of slips.

Even when a slip occurred due to a high traction coefficient caused by gait characteristics such as large step length [26–28], the anterior right edge of the smooth surface component prevented infiltration of the glycerol solution into the contact interface, and the deformation of the tread block increased the contact pressure at the anterior part of the block [29], which allowed the smooth surface part to contact directly with the stainless steel surface (Fig. 8.15b). Therefore, the DCOF reached a high value, resulting in shorter slip distance and slower slip velocity.

In contrast, footwear A, which has the tread blocks with a pear skin-finish surface, has rounded surface asperities. Therefore, the contact pressure between the asperities and the stainless steel floor surface was not high enough to remove the solution film from the

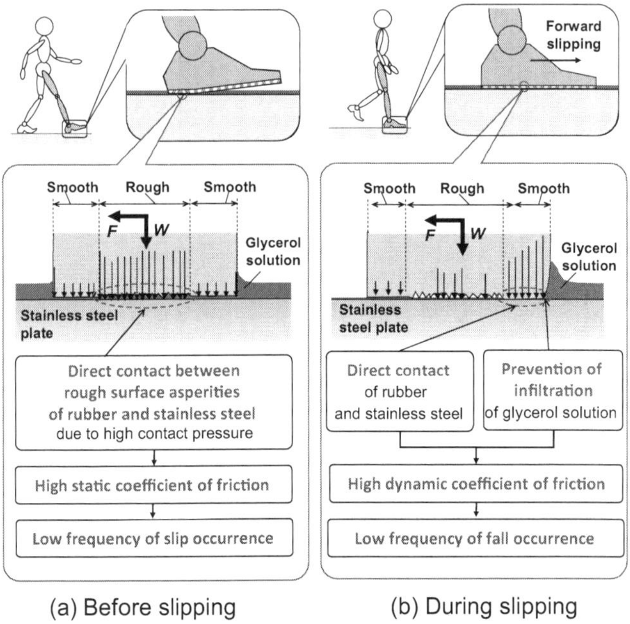

Figure 8.15 Mechanisms of the outsole with the hybrid rubber surface pattern that resulted in low frequencies of the occurrences of slips and falls.

contact interface, which resulted in a low SCOF value when the slip initiated and low DCOF during sliding. Therefore, a slip and fall were more likely to occur for those subjects wearing footwear A compared with those wearing footwear B.

8.5 Conclusion

The hybrid rubber surface pattern with the rough surface area ratio $r = 50\%$ had SCOF and DCOF values greater than 0.4 on a surface covered with a water-based solution. The superior slip resistance of the hybrid rubber surface pattern was achieved by removing the water-based film from the contact interface, resulting in sufficient contact area between the rubber block and surfaces, both when the slip initiated and during sliding. A new footwear sole using the hybrid rubber surface pattern was developed. It was demonstrated that this footwear sole significantly increased slip-resistance on a floor surface contaminated with a water-based solution. The new sole can contribute to the prevention of slipping and falling accidents in work places.

Acknowledgements

The authors would like to thank Kohsin Rubber Co., Ltd. for preparing and providing rubber block specimens and testing footwear. The authors would also like to thank Dr. Hiroshi Onodera at National Hospital Organization CREST laboratory for his excellent help in gait trials and for his valuable comments and suggestions.

References

1. Kawajiri Y, Suzuki Y, Nagata H (2001) Ergonomics studies on analyzing the risk of accidental falls in high-rise construction works. 1. Introduction, *Specif Res Rep Nat Inst Ind Saf*, 22, 1–5.
2. Statistics and Information Department, Minister's Secretariat, Ministry of Health, Labour and Welfare (2011) *Vital statistics of Japan Vol. 3 2009*, Health and Welfare Statistics Association, Japan.
3. Nordin M, Andersson G, Pope M (1997). *Musculoskeletal disorders in the workplace*, Mosby -Year Inc., St Louis.
4. Courtney TK, Sorock GS, Manning DP, Collins JW, Holbein-Jenny MA (2001) Occupational slip, trip, and fall-related injuries–Can the contribution of slipperiness be isolated? *Ergonomics*, 44, 1118–1137.
5. Nagata H, Kim IJ (2009) Fall accidents in Japan and the classification of fall-risk factors, *Proceedings of the International Conference on Slips, Trips, and Falls 2007—From Research to Practice*, 108–112, August 23–24, 2007, Hopkinton, Massachusetts, USA.
6. Grönqvist R (1995) Mechanisms of friction and assessment of slip resistance of new and used footwear soles on contaminated floors, *Ergonomics*, 38, 224–241.
7. Leclercq S, Tisserand M, Saulnier H (1995) Tribological concepts involved in slipping accidents analysis, *Ergonomics*, 38, 197–208.
8. Manning DP, Jones C (2001) The effect of roughness, floor polish, water, oil and ice on underfoot friction: Current safety footwear solings are

less slip resistant than microcellular polyurethane, *Appl Ergon*, 32, 185–196.

9. Grönqvist R, Roine J, Järvinen E, Korhonen E (1989) An apparatus and a method for determining the slip resistance of shoes and floors by simulation of human foot motions, *Ergonomics*, 32, 979–995.
10. Grönqvist R, Hirvonen M, Rajamaki E, Matz S (2003) The validity and reliability of a portable slip meter for determining floor slipperiness during simulated heel strike, *Accid Anal Prev*, 35, 211–225.
11. Redfern MS, Bidanda B (1994) Slip resistance of the shoe–floor interface under biomechanically-relevant conditions, *Ergonomics*, 37, 511–524.
12. Strandberg L (1983) On accident analysis and slip-resistance measurement, *Ergonomics*, 26, 11–32.
13. Fong DTP, Hong Y, Li JX (2009) Human walks carefully when the ground dynamic coefficient of friction drops below 0.41, *Saf Sci*, 47, 1429–1433.
14. Nagata H, Watanabe H, Inoue Y, Kim IJ (2009) Fall and validities of various methods to measure frictional properties of slippery floors covered with soapsuds, *Proceedings of the 17th World Congress on Ergonomics, Beijing, China, 2009*, CD-ROM.
15. Grönqvist R, Hirvonen M, Tohv A (1999) Evaluation of three portable floor slipperiness testers, *Int J Ind Ergon*, 25, 85–95.
16. Wilson M (1990) Development of SATRA slip test and tread pattern design guidelines in *Slips, Stumbles, and Falls: Pedestrian Footwear and Surfaces* (Grey BE, ed) ASTM STP 1103, American Society for Testing and Materials, Philadelphia, 113–123.
17. Chang WR, Kim IJ, Manning DP, Bunterngchit Y (2001) The role of surface roughness in the measurement of slipperiness, *Ergonomics*, 44, 1200–1216.
18. Li KW, Chen CJ (2004) The effect of footwear soling tread groove width on the coefficient of friction with different sole materials, floors, and contaminants, *Appl Ergon*, 35, 499–507.
19. Li KW, Chen CJ (2005) Effects of tread groove orientation and width of the footwear pads on measured friction coefficients, *Saf Sci*, 43, 391–405.
20. Yamaguchi T, Umetsu T, Ishizuka Y, Kasuga K, Ito T, Ishizawa S, Hokkirigawa K (2012) Development of new footwear sole surface pattern for prevention of slip-related falls, *Saf Sci*, 50, 986–994.
21. Yamaguchi T, Kasuga K, Ito T, Ishizawa S, Hokkirigawa K (2012) Development of high grip footwear outsole using hybrid rubber pattern, *Proceedings of NORDTRIB2012*, USB memory.

22. Childs THC, Cowburn D (1984) Contact observations on and friction of rubber drive belting, *Wear*, 100, 59–76.
23. Strandberg L, Lanshammar H (1981) The dynamics of slipping accidents, *J Occup Accid*, 3, 153–162.
24. Brady RA, Pavol MJ, Owings TM, Grabiner MD (2000) Foot displacement but not velocity predicts the outcome of a slip induced in young subjects while walking, *J Biomech*, 33, 803–808.
25. Cham R, Redfern M (2002). Heel contact dynamics during slip events on level and inclined surfaces, *Saf Sci*, 40, 559–576.
26. Yamaguchi T, Hokkirigawa K (2008) "Walking-mode maps" based on slip/non-slip criteria, *Ind Health*, 46, 23–31.
27. Yamaguchi T, Hatanaka S, Hokkirigawa K (2008) Effect of step length and walking speed on traction coefficient and slip between shoe sole and walkway, *Tribol Online*, 3, 59–64.
28. Yamaguchi T, Yamanouchi H, Hokkirigawa K (2008) Experimental analyses of load carrying effects on the peak traction coefficient between shoe sole and floor during walking, *Tribol Online*, 33, 42–347.
29. Besdo D, Heimann B, Klüppel M, Kröger M, Wriggers P, Nackenhorst U (2010) *Elastomere Friction, Theory, Experiment and Simulation*, Springer, Germany.

Index